The Healing Power of Aromatherapy

The Healing Power of Aromatherapy

The Enlightened Person's Guide to the Physical, Emotional, and Spiritual Benefits of Essential Oils

Hasnain Walji, Ph.D.

Prima Publishing

Library of Congress Cataloging-in-Publication Data

Walji, Hasnain.
    The healing power of aromatherapy : the enlightened person's guide to the physical, emotional, and spiritual benefits of essential oils / by Hasnain Walji
        p.   cm.
    Includes biographical references and index.
    ISBN 0-7615-0441-9
    1. Aromatherapy.   I. Title.
    RM666.A68W35   1996
    615'.321—dc20   96-2513
                                                                              CIP

96 97 98 99 00 01 AA 10 9 8 7 6 5 4 3 2 1

Printed in the United States of America

How to Order:

Single copies may be ordered from Prima Publishing, P.O. Box 1260BK, Rocklin, CA 95677; telephone (916) 632-4400. Quantity discounts are also available. On your letterhead, include information concerning the intended use of the books and the number of books you wish to purchase.

To my daughter Sukaina, who is leaving home to sail on the sea of matrimony just as I finish this manuscript.

Contents

Acknowledgments

I would like to express my appreciation to Auriel Mott and David Ponsonby for their dedication and help with the research for this book. I am deeply grateful to Olivier Clerc for assisting me with information from the Scientific Institute of Aromatology (INSA) and C.A.P.M. (Philippe Mailhebiau College of Aromatherapy). I would also like to thank Nadine Artemis and Barbara Collins for their input in dealing with the frequently asked questions (FAQs) on aromatherapy.

Last but not least, I wish to thank my wife, Latifa, for her gentle care and concern, which enabled me to complete this book.

Introduction

For years, aromatherapy was considered unsustainable by many medical and scientific circles, yet it has achieved considerable prominence in Europe, and is currently making steady incursions into the United States. In fact, aromatherapy is not completely new to America. As long ago as 1886, Dr. J. Pemberton (the inventor of Coca-Cola) is reported to have used six essential oils, namely cinnamon, coriander, lemon, neroli, nutmeg, and orange, in his secret flavor formula, 7X.

Recently this seemingly eccentric therapy has become a serious branch of complementary medicine in the United States. Its popularity is amply portrayed in the books and articles that continually appear in the popular press. My sole aim in this book is to simplify the information available and to outline the practical methods of using essential oils as part of a holistic treatment.

I suggest that you acquaint yourself thoroughly with Understanding Essential Oils (page 21) and Aromatherapy in Practice (page 29) to get a good grasp of the subject matter. Other chapters focus on the safe use of essential oils for specific conditions, such as skin care and pregnancy.

The characteristics and therapeutic effects of the commonly used essential oils have been listed alphabetically in the Index of Popular Oils (page 75). The Index of Ailments (page 139) contains brief descriptions for a multitude of conditions, followed by a list of essential oils and their methods of use for those ailments. It is best to refer to the Index of Ailments to identify the most suitable oils and then refer to the Index of Popular Oils for further information on the healing properties and suggested uses of the oils.

Self-treatment with aromatic oils can be a very pleasant experience. Minor burns, stings, headaches, and stress can be managed quite easily as long as you follow the guidelines in this book.

If your condition is one that needs medical attention, or you are pregnant, or the patient is a child, it is best to consult a professional aromatherapist. The

Index of Popular Oils and the Index of Ailments will help you better understand the treatment prescribed by your aromatherapist. An informed patient, as any practitioner will confirm, is a better patient (pun intended) because he or she will be able to take charge of his or her condition and achieve health.

Although most essential oils are quite safe to use for short periods of time, I advise you to consult a practitioner if you intend any extended use. I must also emphasize the preventative nature of aromatherapy and the fact that, in the case of diabetes, cancer, cardiovascular conditions, and other serious illnesses, aromatherapeutic treatment does not obviate the need for proper medical treatment by a medical professional.

Health, as they say, is not just absence of disease. It is positive state of well-being. Aromatherapy can undoubtedly help you achieve that state of well-being. Good health!

The Healing Power of Aromatherapy

An Ancient Therapy
in Modern Times

1

It Pays to Be Scentsible

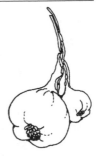

Think back to the last time you ambled through a scented garden. Can you recall the lure of the scented rose, the pungent sweetness of lavender, the dusky aroma of chamomile? Remember how you felt as you drank in the bouquet of smells—content, relaxed, peaceful—you wished you could capture this lovely experience and carry it home with you. This book will explain how to bring the soothing, exhilarating, and enriching benefits of the garden into your own home through the use of plant essences themselves, the essential oils that form the basis of aromatherapy.

As its name suggests, *aromatherapy* (the name given by French chemist Dr. Rene M. Gattefosse in 1928 and meaning "the use of smell to effect a cure") uses the natural scents of plants to heal, to energize , and to relax the body. Aromatherapy heals by stimulating the body's own self-healing powers. It energizes through the selection of particular aromas that wake up our minds and emotions and enable us to move ahead more purposefully. It relaxes us in much the same way—by using one or more essential oils that have calming, sedative properties. These oils are extracted from the parts of the plant that give it its fragrance or flavor—not just the flowers, but also the roots, leaves, seeds, and rinds.

The most common way of applying the essential oils is through massage, usually by a qualified aromatherapist, although techniques can be learned for treatment at home. Other methods of using the oils include bathing, compresses, and scenting rooms—all of which can be undertaken by yourself.

A HOLISTIC THERAPY

Aromatherapy is a healing process that has been designated an "alternative" or "complementary" therapy. When you learn about its ancient foundations, which we'll discuss in the next chapter, you will wonder why it isn't more widely used today, since it has played a dominant role in many major civilizations. However, in common with other alternative therapies, aromatherapy adopts a holistic approach, and it is probably this aspect of it that, in our scientific and skeptical age, has precluded it from achieving its rightful place in our twentieth-century medical systems.

Unlike modern medicine, which tends to look only at the part of the body that is being presented as "ill," which tends to treat symptoms rather than causes, and which tries to suppress those symptoms rather than trying to understand their meaning, holistic therapies aim to treat the whole person.

In holism an individual is seen as mind, soul, and body. Our emotional and mental states can have a bearing on whether we will or will not succumb to a particular illness. It may be, for example, that a person "needs" to be ill. He or she may really be telling the world, "I need looking after." A holistic therapy regards disease as being simply that—a "dis-ease" of the body—and its underlying aim is to find out *why* the individual has become ill and to treat that cause. The illness itself may adversely affect our mind and our feelings. Holistic therapies recognize that the parts of the body are interrelated and that when one part is affected, so are the others. These therapies work with the symptoms, assisting the body in fighting off the infection, which is what the body is actually trying to do, rather than knocking the symptoms on the head, which may leave the body in a still more weakened state, prone to further illness.

Health, in holistic terms, is not simply the absence of disease. It is a positive state of well-being in which all the different elements that make up an individual are in balance and are working in harmony with each other. It follows that the lifestyle of a person is particularly important. Holistic therapies place a great deal of emphasis on correct nutrition, exercise, and mental relaxation, which form the foundation of a healthy body. If an individual eats a healthful (nutrient-rich) diet, exercises regularly, and takes time to relax, there is less likelihood that this individual will succumb to illness, for the body will be better able to stave off an attack from outside.

Nutrition

The holistic approach to nutrition could be summed up by the adage "eat well to be well." Eating well means consuming a diet that is plentiful in all the nutrients needed to build and sustain the growth and repair of the body—proteins, fats, complex carbohydrates, vitamins, and minerals. You can best obtain these by consuming a whole-food diet, which includes whole grains (cereals and breads), a variety of fresh fruits and vegetables, lean meat, chicken, fish, pulses (such as beans and lentils), lowfat dairy products, and eggs. Fresh fruits and some vegetables contain vitamin C, which is particularly important for strengthening the immune system, the health of which is vital if we don't want to fall prey to illness.

In an ideal world none of our foods would be contaminated with the pesticides and herbicides that today's farming methods use to increase crop yield. If you can, try to obtain your foods from organic suppliers.

Exercise

It is well-known that exercise itself can give a real boost to the immune system. It gets blood circulating, helps the body get rid of waste, and can even help us to relax and take our minds off stressful events in our lives.

Try using a reviving blend of cypress, rosemary, and lavender essential oils in a vegetable oil base after you exercise. This makes an ideal muscle-relaxing bath oil, which can be used after any kind of strenuous physical activity.

Relaxation

There are many ways to relax. At its simplest, relaxation may mean going for a walk, listening to your favorite music, or engaging in some other activity that you particularly enjoy, such as gardening or swimming. Other more structured activities include yoga, Tai Chi, and meditation—all these techniques have helped thousands of people to counteract the stresses with which we are all assailed. Of course, massage is another particularly soothing relaxant, especially in conjunction with aromatic essential oils.

Create a relaxing bath oil from a blend of lavender, geranium, and clary sage essential oils in a moisturizing vegetable oil base. This can melt away tension and is the perfect way to prepare for a restful sleep at the end of a long, tiring day.

OTHER PLANT THERAPIES

Aromatherapy is not the only therapy that uses plants for healing—both herbalism and homeopathy base many of their cures on plants and plant extracts. For the purposes of this book, we will concentrate on aromatherapy. However, a brief introduction to these related therapies is in order.

Herbalism

Herbalism's raison d'être is the use of plants for medicinal purposes. Like your own medical practitioner, an herbalist will look at the presenting symptoms. He or she will try to ascertain the chain of events that led up to the problem—whether, for example, there have been any recent emotional stresses such as a change of job, or a bereavement. She or he will also try to find out something about the character of the patient. Is that person highly sensitive; how does the patient respond to life? Past medical history will be discussed, too. The remedy that the herbalist will prescribe will be unique to that particular patient, even though the symptoms may seem identical to another patient's.

The prescribed remedies may take a variety of forms. Unlike the aromatherapy treatments discussed in this book, herbalism often uses treatments administered internally. Infusions (teas) are made from the leaves or flowers or other aerial parts of the plant, which may be fresh or dried. Decoctions are drink preparations that use the woodier parts of the plant, such as the seeds, bark, or roots. These are made by adding boiling water to powdered dried herbs, allowing the brew to simmer for ten to fifteen minutes, and straining it. A capsule containing the powder of ground herbs is another way of administering a dose. Tinctures are concentrated extracts of herbs, which, again, may be either fresh or dried. And some of these remedies may be added to honey or concentrated apple juice or brown sugar to form a syrup.

In addition, herbalists use herbal baths and herbal oils (where the plant is soaked in a vegetable oil that then becomes infused with the properties of that plant). There are creams, ointments, compresses, and poultices. Finally, an herbalist may prescribe an essential oil to be taken by way of a massage, in a bath, or as added to an ointment.

As you can see, herbalism and aromatherapy overlap, and it is possible for the two systems to work together to provide a more complete therapy for the patient.

Homeopathy

The basic principle of homeopathy is that "like cures like." A homeopath, too, will want to take a history of the patient's lifestyle. He or she builds up a picture of that individual's response to mental, emotional, and physical stresses. The patient's strengths and weaknesses are considered and the homeopath tries to determine the patient's underlying constitution. She or he will look at the patient's individual pattern of illness so as to be able to prescribe a precise remedy that matches the particular symptoms the patient is displaying.

Homeopathic remedies differ from those offered by the aromatherapist or herbalist. For example, although many are based on plant material (such as arnica and belladonna), others are derived from minerals (such as sulfur). The other main difference is that the remedies are administered in a very dilute form, thought to be a much gentler way of assisting a cure than the methods prescribed by herbalism. Many homeopaths are of the view that aromatherapy is incompatible with homeopathy; they believe that essential oils can negate or weaken the effects of the homeopathic remedies. Other homeopaths, however, have successfully managed to combine the two.

Bach Flower Remedies

Edward Bach, a consultant bacteriologist and homeopath, developed his flower remedies in the 1930s. They, too, are based on the healing energy of flowering plants and are used to relieve and transform negative emotions, which may be the source of our discomforts. Dr. Bach believed that the properties of thirty-eight flowers could be used to treat all of the known negative mental states. These include such emotions as anger, fear, anxiety, and loss.

In keeping with homeopathic tradition, Bach diluted his remedies, but to a greater degree even than in homeopathy, so that all that is left of the plant is its "trace," its "energy pattern." Needless to say, skepticism has been expressed as to the efficacy of these remedies, but many people can testify to the help that they have received.

ADDRESSING MORE THAN JUST SYMPTOMS

Although aromatherapy adopts a holistic approach to an individual's problems, most people who come to aromatherapy (and, indeed, to the other complementary therapies) do so because they have physical symptoms of illness, and they regard the practitioner much in the same way as they do their doctor. This means that, to some extent, a symptomatic approach cannot be avoided. But a good aromatherapist will prescribe oils that not only address the symptoms but also deal with the underlying cause of the illness (such as stress).

Aromatherapy can be used to treat a wide range of health problems— mental, emotional, and physical. As indicated earlier, aromatherapy can help to counteract the effects of stress, but it can also be used to treat many common ailments, such as bruises, cuts and burns, fungal infections such as athlete's foot, candida albicans (thrush), muscular aches and pains, sore throats, premenstrual syndrome, toothache, and even nosebleeds. It also has been found to be of much benefit for more serious conditions—arthritis and rheumatism, to name but two.

Many people find that the essential oils have helped to improve the condition of their skin and hair. Dermatitis, eczema, and acne can all be treated, as can other less severe complaints such as dry and aging skin, blackheads, broken veins, and greasy skin. Having first been diluted in a carrier oil (see chapter 8) or added to an ointment or cream, the essential oils are applied to the affected areas. A number of cosmetic products on the market are specifically produced according to aromatherapeutic principles. They can usually be purchased from a health food store or by mail order.

Earlier, we mentioned that aromatherapy can be administered in a number of ways, including massage, bathing, compresses, and scenting of rooms. Massage is a very good way of applying essential oils because, apart from the beneficial effects of touch, the effects of the essential oils are immediate. The oils are absorbed through the skin and taken up by the body through the circulation of the blood. This is also true of bathing.

Baths do not have to involve the whole body, however. Hand and foot baths, saunas, inhalation, and facial steaming also are effective. Compresses can be used for injuries and headaches. Certain essential oils make an effective mouthwash or, diluted in water, a pleasant hair rinse. One or two drops placed on a handkerchief can be used for the relief of colds or motion sickness. A few drops of oil added to dried flowers can add fragrance to a room and create a wonderful background against which to work, meditate, or relax, depending on the oils chosen.

Hundreds of essential oils have been identified as having therapeutic properties, but when it comes to deciding which of them to use, an aromatherapist will tend to work with about thirty to treat the most common complaints. If you decide that you want to use the oils yourself at home, whether to treat a condition or to engage in some preventative measures and maintain good health, you may find that your choice of oils also is restricted to those that are most often in demand. However, as more people are becoming aware of the possibilities afforded them by aromatherapy, the range of oils available over-the-counter at most health food stores and at some pharmacies is widening. In chapter 10, you will find a list of the major essential oils with descriptions of their properties and uses. In chapter 11, you will find an index of particular ailments listed with the oils that can be beneficial in treating these conditions. Between the two, you should be able to make an informed decision as to which oils are best suited to your needs.

Dos and Don'ts

Don't take the oils internally.

Don't apply neat (undiluted) essential oils to your skin unless under the supervision of a qualified health care professional.

Do keep oils away from your eyes. If you should accidentally get oil in your eyes, wash them with plenty of water.

Do keep bottles out of reach of small children. Use extra-diluted forms for babies and young children. Use oils for children only under the supervision of a qualified health care professional.

If you are pregnant, *don't* use essential oils except under the supervision of a qualified aromatherapist.

If you suffer from skin allergies, *do* a patch-test before using (see chapter 5).

If you are taking homoeopathic remedies, *do* consult your practitioner before using essential oils.

Don't put essential oils on or near a naked flame. They are flammable.

If you suffer from epilepsy, *do* seek medical advice before using essential oils.

If you are asthmatic, *don't* inhale essential oils.

CAUTIONS

Aromatherapy should *not* be treated as equivalent in value to a beauty therapy. Essential oils should be regarded with the same seriousness and respect as conventional medicines; natural plant substances are drugs and should be recognized as such. Therefore, some aromatherapists are particularly wary of self-administration and self-experimentation and prefer that, for therapeutic purposes, the advice and expertise of a qualified aromatherapist always be sought. Nevertheless, it is recognized that people want to take responsibility for their health and it is also accepted that for minor conditions, self-help can work.

There are circumstances in which extreme caution is urged, particularly if you are pregnant or have a serious health condition or if you are intending to use essential oils on children and infants. In these instances it is wise to consult an aromatherapist. For most people, however, provided you read and adhere to the above list of dos and don'ts you should find nothing but pleasure in your chosen treatment.

This book is intended to provide you with a practical introduction to the healing powers of aromatherapy. We hope that by understanding its principles more thoroughly you will be able to get the best out of essential oils. You may even want to use the book as a starting point for discussions with an aromatherapist. The more knowledgeable you are, the more you can participate in your own health care. It pays to be "scentsible."

2

Magic and Mystery: A Brief History of Aromatherapy

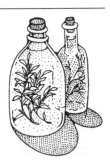

When Dr. Rene Gattefosse introduced the term *aromatherapy* in the early twentieth century he was not describing an innovative method of treatment. The word may have been new, but the practice of aromatherapy has been a part of life since well before recorded history. In fact, it has always been bound up with two of humankind's most basic needs—our dependence on plants for food and medicine, and the expression of our spiritual selves.

ANCIENT EGYPTIANS

Perhaps no other culture understood the interrelationship of these two aspects better than the ancient Egyptians. For them, the magic and mystery of aromatherapy permeated the whole of their daily existence. We know from records dating back to around 4500 B.C. that their practice of medicine, rituals, embalming, and astrology incorporated the use of fragrant spices and oils, resins and bark, and that their vinegars, wines, and beers were scented.

Other sources describe the particular blends of sweet-smelling substances that were used by the priests and alchemists to make perfumes and medicines. Some of the perfumes were used in rituals to heighten religious experience and fervor. *Kyphi* is one of these. This preparation included sixteen separate aromatic ingredients, among them saffron, juniper, myrrh, cassia, spikenard, and cinnamon. During important festivals the city squares exuded the aromas of burning piles of fragrant substances.

We also know that, for medicinal purposes, plants and their properties were relied on to treat a wide range of conditions. The prescribed remedy for hay fever, for instance, was a mixture of antimony (a silvery white chemical compound), aloe, myrrh, and honey. As a contraceptive measure, a combination of acacia, coloquinte (a bitter-apple pulp), dates, and honey was placed in the vagina to ferment into lactic acid. We now know that lactic acid acts as a spermicide.

Foods, too, were infused with fragrances that helped the digestive processes. Caraway, coriander, and aniseed were added to bread. Onions and garlic, with their stimulating and antibacterial properties, formed a staple part of the diet. Garlic was given to the slaves who built the pyramids to ensure that sickness did not interfere with the important job of building a tomb for their pharaoh.

We are all aware of the Egyptians' mummification of their dead. The embalmers of those times used the preservative properties of plants to ensure the safe arrival of the deceased into the next world. Cedarwood and myrrh were highly prized in this process, but other plants with antiseptic and antibacterial qualities were also part of the embalmer's repertoire, including cinnamon, cloves, nutmeg, and resins such as galbanum. It is reported that when the tomb of Tutankhamen was opened in 1922, the odors of the preservatives used were still detectable, and pots were found containing myrrh and frankincense.

The fame of the Egyptian priests and priestesses spread far and wide and many physicians and wise men from other cultures made the pilgrimage to Egypt to learn from them. Also famous were the Egyptian botanical gardens, which contained plants brought from as far away as China and India.

The oils that the ancient Egyptians used were extracted in two main ways. The first involved the process of distillation. Large clay pots were filled first with plant material and then with water. The neck of the pot was stopped up with woolen fibers and the pot was heated. The steam carried the essential oils upward where they were trapped by the wool. The fibers were then squeezed to release the oils. The other method of extraction involved gathering the flowers into a large cloth bag with sticks attached to it. The sticks were twisted around and around until the oils were squeezed out of the petals.

Some archeologists believe that the ancient Egyptians obtained their oils in yet another way, by the process of infusion. The plants were left in the sun for a few days, sitting on top of a layer of oil or fat. These bases would then take on the aromas of the plant material. But whatever method was used, it can be said that the ancient Egyptians were the first true aromatherapists.

THE CHINESE

Separately, but no less importantly, the Chinese were developing their own system of herbal medicine. In fact, the earliest written herbal reference book was compiled by the emperor Shen Nung. *The Great Herbal,* or *Pen Tsao,* is thought to date back to between 1000 and 700 B.C. and contains references to at least 350 medicinal plants and remedies.

Much of the ancient Chinese use of herbal medicine was in conjunction with acupuncture and massage. But their alchemists also were concerned with finding the key to immortality through experimentation with plant perfumes, which, they believed, contained magical forces and the spirits of plants. The homes of the wealthy included an *artemisia room,* a room set aside especially for childbirth. During labor the artemisia plant was burned to encourage the presence of friendly spirits and to help relax the mother and her baby.

THE GREEKS AND ROMANS

The next major civilization to recognize the central importance of herbal medicine and its aromatic principles was Greek. The Greeks were much influenced by the Egyptians. As in Egypt, the Greeks burned incense in their holy places and in the city squares. Homes often had a small shrine where the gods could be placated by incense. Clothing, foods, and wine were scented, too— perhaps with myrrh, rose, and violet.

Hippocrates developed herbal medicine into a more scientific discipline, basing the prescription of a medicine upon accurate observation and diagnosis. He believed in the importance of daily aromatic baths and massage to maintain health and preserve life. When the plague broke out in Athens, he exhorted the populace to burn aromatic plants on street corners to prevent the plague from spreading. The knowledge of botany was also being extended at this time; Theophrastus, considered the "father of botany," wrote his masterpiece, the *Historia Plantarum.*

The Greeks and the Egyptians greatly influenced the therapeutic use of plants by the Roman civilization. The Romans laid great store by the culinary potential of plants (they introduced the seeds of many of their favorite herbs into other parts of Europe as their legions advanced), but it was the Greek physician Dioscorides, a surgeon in Nero's army, and his fellow Greek physicians and thinkers who influenced the Roman sphere of medicine. Dioscorides wrote *De Materia Medica,* an encyclopedia of medical plants and their properties. His observations as to when the active principles of plants are at their height are still relied on today by the harvesters of essential oils. The active principles of a poppy, for example, are much greater in the morning than at any other time of the day. It was Dioscorides who first cured pain by using a decoction of willow, the source of aspirin. The Egyptian influence on the Romans is evident from the prominence given to aromatic baths and massage.

THE ARABS

The importance of Arab contributions to medicine and scientific inquiry should not be underestimated. From about the fourth century their civilization developed rapidly. They were extraordinary explorers and travelers, venturing as far afield as Russia and Sweden and the Far East, and it was they who introduced many of the plants and spices so familiar to us today—sandalwood, cloves, nutmeg, camphor, and cassia—for use in medicines, perfumes, and cooking.

Abu Ibn Sina (known in the West as Avicenna), the famous Muslim physician, philosopher, astronomer, and mathematician, is credited with inventing the process of distillation of essential oils, the principles of which are the basis for extraction even now. Avicenna was also the author of a medical textbook, the *Canon of Medicine*. Written in the eleventh century, it was referred to right up until the middle of the sixteenth century.

THE MIDDLE AGES AND RENAISSANCE IN EUROPE

In Europe during the Middle Ages, monasteries and religious communities kept learning alive and were the repository of knowledge about plants and their healing powers. The Norman conquerors brought with them the custom of strewing aromatic plants on the ground to fragrance their surroundings, to combat such pests as fleas and lice, and to ward off disease. In the twelfth century the Crusaders returned from their exploits, bringing back with them oils, perfumes, and the knowledge of distillation, which they had learned from the Arabs. St. Hildegarde of Bingen, a thirteenth-century abbess, was particularly knowledgeable, and her four treatises on the medicinal properties of plants are still referred to.

In the early fourteenth century, when the black death swept across Europe, people were told to carry aromatic pomanders and to burn aromatic substances in the houses and on street corners; nevertheless, about one-third to one-half of the population of Europe was wiped out. One striking fact is that the rate of survival of the perfumers during the plague was high.

The Renaissance, beginning in the fifteenth century, saw a revival of the spirit of discovery. Christopher Columbus and Vasco de Gama made their dangerous expeditions, bringing back from their travels new plants from the American continent, such as coca leaves and balsams used by the Incas and the North American Indians respectively.

HERBAL MEDICINE MEETS MODERN SCIENCE

In Britain, in the sixteenth and seventeenth centuries, herbal medicine reached its peak of influence with the publication of a number of herbals, some by practitioners whose names still inspire awe—Thomas Culpeper and Charles Gerard. From that time onward scientific inquiry really took off, with new discoveries that were to change the face of medicine forever. Chemists were learning how to isolate the active principles within plants and to manufacture them synthetically. The prevailing belief was that the other constituents of plants were unnecessary and even impure and should be discarded. Such was the faith in the new medicine that, by the nineteenth century, herbal remedies and essential oils were regarded as belonging to the realms of superstition and folk tradition, as little more than the "magic" of primitive peoples.

GATTEFOSSE REKINDLES INTEREST IN ESSENTIAL OILS

Truths have a way of reasserting themselves, however. It was a chance incident that rekindled interest in the healing powers of essential oils. Rene Gattefosse was a French chemist who worked in his family's perfumery business. Although the essential oils were being used exclusively for cosmetic purposes, his observations led him to appreciate their antiseptic qualities. One day, while working in his laboratory, he burned his hand severely in an explosion. Immediately he plunged his hand into some lavender essence that happened to be nearby. To his amazement, the burn healed very quickly, without infection or scarring. As a result, Gattefosse turned his scientific attention to the medical properties of essential oils and their beneficial effects on skin conditions.

During the First World War, he tried out essential oils on patients in military hospitals and obtained impressive results using such oils as chamomile, thyme, and lemon. These were documented in his book *Aromatherapie*, which was well received by other experts who went on to do their own research. Professor Paolo Rovesti, Director of the Instituto Derivati Vegatali in Milan, for example, was able to show that depression and anxiety could be relieved by the inhalation of the oils from certain plants. Rovesti believed that these smells helped to bring to the surface repressed emotions and memories, which were contributing to the ill health of his patients.

Another French doctor can be credited with consolidating the practice of aromatherapy for medical purposes. Dr. Jean Valnet was an ex-army surgeon who, during the Second World War, used essential oils for treating wounded soldiers. Up until that time, too, essential oils of clove, lemon, thyme, and chamomile were used to fumigate hospital wards, as natural disinfectants, and to sterilize surgical instruments. Valnet also found that he was able to cure long-term psychiatric patients by administering essential oils internally, with, in some cases, almost immediate results. Dr. Valnet also wrote a book entitled *Aromatherapie*, which has been translated into English as *The Practice of Aromatherapy*.

The popular image of aromatherapy can be attributed to the biochemist Marguerite Maury. It was she who linked the use of essential oils with massage. She also must be credited with the concept of choosing and mixing particular oils to suit the needs of individual clients, thereby introducing the holistic approach to the therapy. While treating her clients for cosmetic problems, Maury discovered that their skin disorders not only cleared, but they experienced pleasurable side effects such as improved sleep, reduced symptoms of rheumatism, and increased mental alertness. Some of these benefits continued to be felt weeks and even months after the cessation of treatment.

In Europe, aromatherapy and herbalism (known as phytotherapy) are practiced conjointly by many doctors, and it is generally recognized that the "magic and mystery" of essential oils is based on observable scientific fact. In Britain and North America, on the other hand, there is still a considerable degree of skepticism as to the efficacy of aromatherapy and it continues to be relegated to the realms of "alternative" therapies, with all that that implies.

3

The Philosophy of
Holistic Healing

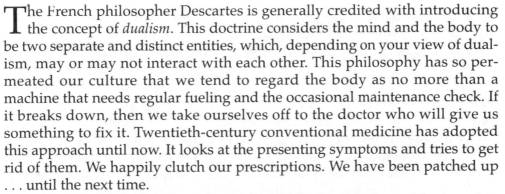

The French philosopher Descartes is generally credited with introducing the concept of *dualism*. This doctrine considers the mind and the body to be two separate and distinct entities, which, depending on your view of dualism, may or may not interact with each other. This philosophy has so permeated our culture that we tend to regard the body as no more than a machine that needs regular fueling and the occasional maintenance check. If it breaks down, then we take ourselves off to the doctor who will give us something to fix it. Twentieth-century conventional medicine has adopted this approach until now. It looks at the presenting symptoms and tries to get rid of them. We happily clutch our prescriptions. We have been patched up . . . until the next time.

But some people seem to take an awful lot of patching up. They are forever at the doctor's clinic with some complaint or other. Such people may come to be viewed as hypochondriacs, people who invent illnesses or believe themselves to be worse than they really are. Or, if they are exhibiting genuine symptoms, these may be termed *psychosomatic* and not taken seriously. And here lies a conundrum, for if these patients really are using their minds to create their illnesses, how can it then be said that the body and the mind are separate and distinct? One is surely influencing the other. And if it is the mind that is making these patients ill, would it not make more sense to treat the mind rather than the body, so that the real problem is being addressed?

It is becoming increasingly obvious, even to the medical establishment, that disease and illness are much more complicated than they appear and involve the interplay of a myriad of factors. For why does one person come down with an illness when another, who may have been exposed to the same conditions, does not? Why do some patients with terminal diseases, such as cancer, succumb while others go into remission? We've all heard stories about individuals who have refused to give in to their illness and who have triumphed against all odds. When confronted with these anomalies we are forced to reassess our views on health and disease and to acknowledge that, perhaps, the physical and the ethereal are bound up with each other more than we had previously realized. A comforting bedside manner, for example, may be the real reason for the cure, rather than any medication that might have been administered.

SEPARATION OF MIND AND BODY—A FALSE PREMISE

Holistic practitioners have long recognized that the separation of mind and body is a false premise and that a great deal of our suffering is attributable to more than our body parts simply wearing out. In holistic therapy the person is viewed as a whole being and it is impossible to say where the body ends and the mind begins. Underlying reasons for an illness have to be considered if there is to be any true healing.

The holistic practitioner will look for the meaning behind the illness. What are these symptoms saying about the individual? What does he want out of his life that he isn't getting? What is his attitude toward life? Are there recurring patterns in his illnesses? Has there been a major life change that renders him emotionally, and therefore physically, more vulnerable to attack?

Or maybe the illness is the body's way of making us stop and think, of giving us the chance to set aside the more immediate concerns of living and to evaluate what we actually want out of life. Here, the body may be telling the mind that we're heading in the wrong direction. Sometimes the body might become ill just to take our minds off the problems that beset us. We become so engrossed in the physical discomforts that we set aside the more important, but seemingly insoluble, matters for a while. In this way we free the mind to come up with its own solution in its own time. Worrying a problem to death may produce just that result, and being ill may actually prevent us from undergoing an untimely demise.

The interconnectedness of the mind and body can easily be seen when you look at your physical reactions to a thought or a feeling or look at the thought or feeling that results from a physical sensation. Messages from our minds to our bodies, or vice versa, involve many systems within the body—the bloodstream, nervous system, and a number of hormones that are secreted by the endocrine glands. All of these systems are regulated by the pituitary gland and the hypothalamus, which is a small region of the brain.

Body functions, e.g. heartbeat and temperature, are kept going by the hypothalamus, which is a bit like the operations room of an electricity grid, with nerve fibers from all over the brain linking into it. This is how the connections are made between the way the body functions and the emotions. If, for example, we are suffering from stress or anxiety, this may manifest itself in disorders of the stomach.

The vegas nerve runs directly between the hypothalamus and the stomach. Other nerves run between the hypothalamus and the thymus and spleen, which play vital roles in our physical health since they are part of the immune system, manufacturing the blood cells that resist outside invaders and controlling immunity in the blood. Feelings of anxiety and fear result in the release of adrenaline, which then circulates, preparing us to fight or flee. In so doing, adrenaline interferes with the messages between the brain and the immune system so that the system starts to shut down, thereby lowering our resistance to disease. Indeed, many negative emotions, if not allowed to be expressed and gotten out of our system, will have a similar effect.

The hypothalamus sits within the limbic area of the brain. This system regulates such bodily processes as the balancing of our bodily fluids, the secretions of the endocrine system, and gastrointestinal activity. Its other main function is to draw together our emotions, which are then linked with our endocrine and hormone systems. The hypothalamus receives its messages from the cerebral cortex of the brain, which has responsibility for thinking, memory, perception, and interpretation. It also receives messages from the olfactory nerves in our noses.

AROMA AND EMOTIONAL WELL-BEING

Research is beginning to show just how important aroma is to our emotional well-being and state of health. Pleasant (and not-so-pleasant) smells can trigger a memory. If the memory is one that we cherish or recall with fondness, such as the scent of a log fire, the odor of an apple pie baking in the oven, or a partner's favorite scent, we feel warm and uplifted and able to meet the challenges that come our way. Unpleasant smells usually evoke unhappy memories, ones that perhaps we would prefer to keep suppressed. Some examples are the odors of sewage, dog waste, diesel fumes (Dodd and Skinner 1992; Wildwood 1991). Of course, aromatherapists also are aware that unpleasant experiences occurring in conjunction with a normally "pleasant" smell can make that scent distasteful to the affected individual. That is why a good aromatherapist will always test a client's reaction to an oil before using it.

Through the use of EEGs (electroencephalographs) to monitor brainwaves, it has been possible to actually see what is happening when a smell is being perceived. A state of mental alertness has been observed when the individual is breathing in such aromas as peppermint, rosemary, and basil. Not only are more beta waves (typical of a state of mental alertness) produced, but subjects are also more accurate in performing tasks set for them than those who do not breathe in scented air (Paleologos 1990; Wildwood 1991).

Other fragrances elicit more alpha, theta, and delta waves. These waves indicate a more relaxed and meditative state of mind. For those who find it difficult to fall asleep or who experience poor sleep, these findings are encouraging. Researchers who monitored subjects for brain waves, heart rate, and sleeping stages found that odors could be perceived during sleep and that fragrances did have a relaxing effect on their subjects. Spiced apple, for example, has been clinically proven to reduce the effects of stress by helping to lower blood pressure (Paleologos 1990).

The essential oil of juniper is thought to release hormones that, in turn, facilitate water loss—of benefit to those who suffer from water retention. Chamomile stimulates the formation of endorphins (the body's natural pain killers) and thus can help to relieve pain. Apart from encouraging mental alertness and, possibly, enhancing the learning process, rosemary has been found to stir up memories (James 1990). This is particularly important for illnesses that may be the expression of years of repressed emotions. Once these emotions are released, through stimulation by such an essential oil, healing can begin. It is thought that some essential oils may help the immune system to function more effectively. The more resistant we are to infection, the more energy we feel and the more we are able to cope with what life throws at us.

Surprisingly, babies have a highly developed sense of smell; they are able to distinguish between odors that we adults cannot (Paleologos 1990). It seems that as we get older we lose some of our sensitivity to smell. However, studies at Warwick University in England have discovered that our skin can respond to odors of which we are entirely unaware. In one experiment, individuals were exposed to the sex pheromone that is excreted in boar's urine. Although most of the subjects could not even smell it, clear skin responses were detected by the EEG machine (Ryan 1988).

We also have the capacity to block the effect of an aroma if we find it repugnant, which is why it is better in aromatherapy to go with the nose rather than to choose an essential oil for its chemical properties only (Wildwood 1991). Researchers at the University of Warwick are attempting to produce a fragrant sponge that will promote tranquillity and reduce reliance on sedative drugs. There are also plans for a fragrant sponge that will suppress the appetite (First Annual International Conference on the Psychology of Perfumery 1986).

The medical establishment is latching onto the benefits of pleasant aromas in other ways. Patients who have to undergo diagnostic imaging scans are often terrified of the noisy machinery that surrounds them and in which they have to lie very still for long periods. If the patient becomes very frightened, the scan may have to be disrupted, at great financial cost. At the Sloan-Kettering Cancer Center in New York steps are being taken to ease the discomfort. They are administering the synthetic scent of the heliotrope flower to the patient through a nasal respirator and are finding that the effect on the patient is a soothing one (*Medical* Update 1991).

Business, too, is taking notice of the research, having discovered that employees who work with a background of aromatic fragrances have enhanced mental states. Some offices, particularly in Japan, have a separate relaxation room to which their workers can retire if they need an energy boost (Paleologos 1990).

The perfume industry has the most to gain financially from scientific inquiry and it will come as no surprise to learn that in 1982 a fund was established by the Fragrance Foundation to provide grants for research projects into the psychology of fragrance—how smell affects human behavior. What is becoming evident from the research is that the body's response to synthetic smells and to natural fragrances is quite different, even though the difference may not be detectable by the nose (James 1990). This is important for the consumer because the trend now is to choose fragrances that have an effect on the wearer rather than on others. People want a fragrance that will make them feel glad to be alive. Pure essential oils are the only fragrances that can ensure that exactly the right messages of well-being are being sent to the brain. For the perfume industry this means a return to natural sources if they want to sell their products.

Touch Is Essential for Health

One of the most important developments in modern aromatherapy has been the greater emphasis on massage. Surely there can be no better example of the interconnectedness of mind and body, for in the touching there is a physical relaxation that results in a mental and emotional release.

It is well-known that touch is essential for good health. As babies our lives depend on it. Touch forms a part of the important process of bonding after birth. The fondling, kissing, cuddling, and carrying of the baby helps her or him to form relationships and to integrate into society. A baby who receives little such attention may fail to thrive—quite literally feel that life isn't worth living, shut down his or her survival mechanisms, and become ill. But all is not lost if the initial bonding process is impaired, for whatever reason. By increasing skin contact—through massage, cuddling, rocking, and holding—parents can make up for lost time. Research on premature babies has found that those infants who received massage from their mothers had better nerve and brain cell development. They gained weight faster and were generally healthier (Stanway 1987).

This need to be touched remains with us throughout our lives, even though we as adults may try to ignore it. It is the medium through which love is communicated and is the basis for massage. It is very important, therefore, that you feel able to surrender yourself into the hands of your masseur or masseuse. His or her empathy creates the environment that will enable the treatment to have maximum effect.

In physical terms, what appears to happen during massage is that the receptor nerves in the skin are stimulated to send messages to the brain. These messages, in turn, stimulate the brain to send messages back to the same zones in the body that are being massaged. The voluntary muscles in those areas relax, the blood capillaries open and close, and nerve sensors may become sedated, bringing about relief from pain. Over time these effects can bring about changes in the organs to which those zones relate. The relaxation that massage engenders frees the body to get on with the important tasks of self-healing and repair; it frees the mind by relieving us, for a time, of our mental baggage.

By combining aroma and touch, aromatherapy can meet some of our most basic needs. Through the use of therapeutic essential oils and skilled manipulation, deep-seated emotions can be released, and this can have an important bearing on our long-term health (Shapiro 1990). Individuals who repress their emotions for fear of what others think, who have a tendency toward depression, and who turn in on themselves are at a greater risk of developing cancer. This fact alone makes it clear just how much aromatherapy has to offer for total healing.

4

Understanding Essential Oils: How They Work and How to Buy Them

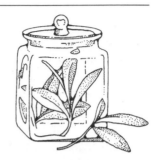

Human beings are complex. We function on many different levels—from our most basic physical requirements to the many social and emotional interactions we experience with other people. All these different aspects of ourselves have been placed within two distinct categories—"mind" and "body." Some (particularly those with a religious view of humankind) would add a third—the "spirit."

In holism, all these elements combine to make up one distinct and unique individual. When it comes to true healing, all these parts of the whole must be taken into account. Essential oils also are complex and, as you have seen, can address the needs of the whole person. They are truly fitting remedies for our time.

How Do Essential Oils Exert Their Effects?

Oils exert their effects in two ways. The first is through absorption through the skin. If you rub a clove of garlic on the soles of your feet, its odor can be detected on your breath a few hours later. What better proof that, far from being impermeable, the skin is actually able to take in substances. Modern science is recognizing this capacity of the body's largest organ and is using it to advantage. Some drugs are now being administered through skin patches— estrogen, for example, for hormone replacement therapy in women, and nicotine for those people who are trying to give up smoking.

Gattefosse was able to show that although water and watery substances find it difficult to pass through the skin, fats can do so if the molecules are small enough. The molecules of essential oils are believed to enter the skin through the openings of the hair follicles, mix with the natural oily secretions of the skin (sebum), and then find their way either into the bloodstream or into the lymph and interstitial fluid that surrounds all the cells of the body.

You can see just how pervasive and deeply acting the aroma molecules are. Depending on how much subcutaneous fat the individual has, the process of absorption can take anywhere from a few minutes to several hours. This facility of the skin is why modern aromatherapy relies so heavily on massage; aromatic baths; or, sometimes, the application of the oils neat (undiluted).

The second way in which essential oils enter the body is through our air passages. When we breathe in an aroma, the molecules in that aroma are inhaled. Once they reach the lungs, they pass through the air sacs into the blood capillaries and then into the bloodstream, where they circulate.

Not only do the oils work at the most basic level in the body, but they also are effective because they are each made up of different chemical components, perhaps up to a hundred, in varying amounts. In other words, a single essential oil is composed of a variety of molecules that interact with and counterbalance each other. This is why synthetically produced substances can never entirely replicate the natural original and why, sometimes, an individual can have an adverse reaction to a synthetic product. The other elements of the natural substance are not there to keep the active principle in check.

Take lemongrass oil as one example. Its major constituent is an aldehyde citral, which accounts for 80 percent of its chemical components. If the citral is extracted on its own or is chemically synthesized, it causes an allergic response when applied to skin. Lemongrass oil itself, however, does not have this effect, and testing has shown that the other 20 percent of its constituents neutralize the potentially harmful effects of the citral.

This does not mean that essential oils cannot have adverse effects. As a general rule, however, the other constituents of a natural essential oil render the toxin less hazardous. When mixed with other essential oils by an experienced aromatherapist, the toxin is not only diluted still further but the new combination enhances and modifies the effects of all the ingredients of each oil.

When aromatic oils are inhaled, the effects are mediated not just through the absorption of the molecules through the lungs. We mentioned earlier that things that smell (pleasant or unpleasant) give off molecules. When these are inhaled, and while they are embarking on their journey to the lungs, some of them dissolve in the mucus in our noses and meet the olfactory cells, which are located in the upper part of the nose within the mucous membrane. These cells are highly specialized. Each is connected to the brain by a nerve fiber. At the membrane end of the cell is a tiny protrusion of hairlike structures that are especially sensitive to smell. When the molecule hits the cell after having been dissolved in the mucus, a message is passed immediately through the nerve fiber to the olfactory area of the brain, which is closely connected with the limbic area.

You will recall that the limbic area is involved in our emotional responses, memory, sex drive, and intuition. The olfactory area is also connected to the hypothalamus and the pituitary gland, which control the hormones of the nervous and endocrine systems. Experts now believe that the same genes that control our sense of smell are also responsible for controlling the body's ability to distinguish between "self" and "non-self" invaders and thus affect the status of the immune system. Essential oils work on these systems of the body to produce the desired mental and emotional effect.

Essential oils also work on the physical body. Recall from chapter 2 how the founders of modern aromatherapy used essential oils to treat patients with burns, war wounds, and skin conditions, and how essential oils were used to disinfect hospital wards. Tea tree oil, for example, is a more powerful antiseptic than carbolic acid. Bergamot, chamomile, and lavender oil also are natural antiseptics. Chamomile is believed to be 120 times more antiseptic than saltwater.

Methods of Extraction

It is important that the essential oils used, either by an aromatherapist or by oneself at home, contain all of their natural constituents, for otherwise you are wasting your money. While the oil you purchase may smell pleasant, it may be so adulterated that it has no actual therapeutic properties. Whether an oil retains or loses these depends on how the oil has been extracted.

As we discussed in chapter 2, the ancient Egyptians are thought to have had two main methods of obtaining the essential oils. One was through the process of steam distillation—they filled a clay pot with plant material, covered it with water, stopped up the neck of the pot with fibers, and then heated the pot so that the steam containing the essential oil was trapped in the fibers, which were later squeezed. The other method was to squeeze the oil from flowers within a material bag. Today essential oils are often extracted using steam distillation, a modern variation of the former Egyptian technique. The plant material is sometimes combined with water and after it has been heated, the steam passes into a condenser and then into a separator.

Alternatively, rather than the plant material being in direct contact with the water, it may be distilled by the steam itself, which passes over or through the plant material and collects the essential oils on the way. (This is the technique that was devised by Avicenna in the eleventh century.) The possibility of the plants being burned is thereby avoided. A more recent enhancement of this technique is vacuum distillation. The distillation equipment is sealed and the air pressure inside it is reduced, thereby creating a vacuum. This enables the aromas to be more easily preserved since distillation takes place at much lower temperatures.

Oils from citrus fruits are extracted by *expression,* a method that involves squeezing or using pressure. This once was done by hand but is now commonly performed through applying centrifugal force by machine.

At this point it should be mentioned that there is a difference between a plant essence and the essential oil derived from the plant. Sometimes the words are used interchangeably, but chemically they are different substances. An *essence* comes from the plant's reproductive organs and is a natural aromatic substance. An *essential oil,* however, is a distilled essence and the process of distillation causes changes in the nature and composition of the essence.

There has been some concern that modern mechanical techniques, while undoubtedly helping to increase yields and also reducing production costs, may affect the therapeutic value of the oils themselves. This is particularly the case when volatile solvents are used to extract plant oils. The results of such extraction are known as *concretes.* This process is used more by the perfume industry, since it enables the full aroma to be captured, but would never be used by an aromatherapist, because the solvents not only affect the constituents of the oils but they also introduce unwanted chemical residues.

The technique used in solvent extraction is similar to steam distillation. The plant matter is placed on racks in tanks. The volatile solvents are heated and then pass through the racks, taking up the essential oils on the way. Subsequently, the solvents are evaporated off leaving behind the fragrance— and the solvent residues. The solvents used include petroleum ether, hexane, and benzene. The last is being used less frequently, however, since it has been found to cause allergies.

In the perfume industry, plant extracts can go through one more process. A concrete can be refined still further to produce an *absolute,* in which alcohol is added to the concrete. Some of the constituents of the extract dissolve into the alcohol. The alcohol is then evaporated off, leaving behind a substance, the absolute, which has now been even more chemically altered. Sometimes plant material is dissolved directly in alcohol, particularly resinous matter and gums such as myrrh and frankincense. Again the alcohol is evaporated off, leaving behind a heavy, sticky substance. The cosmetics industry makes much use of these products in soaps, creams, shampoos, and, of course, perfumes.

Other techniques of extraction are being investigated, however. One method that may be of benefit to aromatherapy is carbon dioxide extraction, because it does not leave chemical residues. However, the cost is currently high and it remains to be seen whether there are any latent disadvantages to this method.

CONCERNS ABOUT OTHER CHEMICAL RESIDUES

Modern extraction methods are not the only aspects of essential oil cultivation that are causing some aromatherapists anxiety. As with all aspects of twentieth-century farming, questions are being asked about the effects that pesticides and fertilizers are having on the composition of the chemicals in the plants which are used in therapy, whether in aromatherapy or in herbal medicine. Residues of nitrates have been detected in plant oils. We all know, too, about nuclear fallout, acid rain, and pollution—all of which may compromise the purity of the oils. Perhaps purchasers of an oil can do little about the large-scale environmental problems that beset growers, but they can take some steps to ensure that the oils they buy are as pure as they can be.

BUYER BEWARE

To begin with, you can try to ensure that the oils have been extracted from organically grown plants. Unfortunately, it is not always easy to find suppliers of such oils because there are so few of them, and the range of oils they provide may be somewhat limited. Also, while the oils themselves may have been grown organically, it is still possible for a deception to be perpetrated on the unsuspecting purchaser. One example given by Daniele Ryman in her book *Aromatherapy* is lavender. To the uninitiated, lavender, lavandin, and aspic have the same smell (lavandin is a hybrid—a cross between lavender and aspic, which has a stronger smell but fewer therapeutic qualities). Lavandin is frequently marketed as lavender because it is much cheaper. Another possible deception is dilution, perhaps by adding a vegetable oil or a similar smelling oil (lavandin could be added to lavender, for example).

Establishing Standards of Quality

In order to prevent such abuses, moves are afoot to introduce some mark of quality or to have the bottles labeled. The Essential Oil Trade Association

UK is trying to ensure that only pure, unadulterated oils are marketed for aromatherapeutic purposes. Such oils would be stamped with the mark of such organizations as the Soil Association in the UK or the IFOAM (International Federation of Organic Agricultural Movements). In France the problem is being addressed by the Scientific Institute of Aromatology (INSA). This organization includes experts from a broad range of disciplines who are particularly knowledgeable about plants, plant essences, and essential oils.

These doctors, biologists, agronomists, and pharmacists research developing the quality of essential oils and how that quality can be controlled. They believe that it is vital to know the origin of the essential oil and that such origin should itself be certified to show that it meets a required standard. They propose a certificate that would be awarded to the particular producer who has reached that standard, a plan that has now been established. Known as the HEBBD (Huile Essentielle Botaniquement et Biochimiquement Definie, Botanically and Biochemically Defined Essential Oil), the certificate defines three criteria that should be disclosed by the producer about his or her product: (1) the botanical name, (2) which plants were distilled, and (3) environmental specificities (climate, soil, season of harvest, etc.) that might affect the chemical compositition of the plant.

Look for Botanical Names

The INSA prefers the retention of the Latin botanical names since this leads to fewer errors in classification. In France, for example, the word *citronelle* is used to describe a variety of plants that give off a warm lemony smell. These could include *Cymbopogon nardus* (Ceylon citronella), *Cymbopogon winterianus* (Java citronella), and *Cymbopogon citratus* (lemongrass) or even other lemony-scented plants from completely different families, such as *Melissa officinalis* (lemon balm, melissa, lamiaceae) and *Lippia citriodora* (verbena). Furthermore, unless the labeling is complete, purchasers may be confused as to the true nature of the oil and why the expected results do not occur. Just because one oil has the same smell as another does not mean that it has the same therapeutic properties.

The INSA also warns us to be on guard against oils that do not actually exist. You may find an oil on the shelves labeled "hawthorn." But it is impossible to distill the essence of hawthorn, which means that any such oil being sold has been synthetically produced using anisic aldehyde, which is hawthorn's main constituent.

What Part of the Plant Has Been Distilled?

The second criterion that the INSA believes should be mentioned on the label is which particular part of the plant has been distilled, especially for aromatic trees and shrubs. The therapeutic value of the oil often depends upon whether it has been extracted from the flowers or the leaves or the peel. *Citrus aurantium var. amara* (one of the orange family) is valued for the oil that is derived from its flowers (Neroli), from the leaves (bitter orange leaf), and from the peel of the fruit (zest essence), all of which have significantly different properties.

Biochemical Specificities

Finally, the INSA wants information included about such factors as climate, soil conditions, altitude, and latitude. They describe these influences as *biochemical specificities* that affect the genetic makeup of the plant and give it its individual characteristics. These specificities will affect the chemical composition of the plant and thus its therapeutic action.

The season in which a plant is harvested also makes a difference. These seasonal variations in the chemical components of plant essences enable the plant to cope with adverse conditions. This helps to explain why wild plant essences are more therapeutically beneficial than cultivated ones.

Daniele Ryman believes that one other item of information that should be recorded is the date of distillation. An oil that has sat on the shelves for too long can sometimes cause an allergic reaction in an individual.

Although certain elements of oils defy identification and it is still not fully understood how all the chemical components interact with each other to produce a therapeutic result, the more information consumers have regarding the oil, the better they will be able to make an informed judgment.

Another Method of Chemical Analysis

Another method to ensure that the oils are authentic is to analyze them using gas chromatography linked to a mass spectrometer, a technique used by laboratories, scientists, and manufacturers for quality control. In this way it is possible to see depicted in graph form each of the chemical compounds that makes up the aromatic substance. This method of analysis has been likened to the "fingerprint" of an essential oil. The fingerprint (chromatographic profile) can then be compared with other chromatographic profiles that have been made of other samples of essential oils.

From the comparison with the original profile it should be possible to detect whether a fraud is being perpetrated. The profile will show whether an oil has been adulterated by, for example, the mixing of two oils of close or different compositions, or whether it contains traces of solvents or mineral oils. If it does, then it is obviously not a pure essential oil.

Shopping Smart

Until rigorous testing is carried out on all essential oils, and until certification or labeling of one sort or another is established, the best way to ensure that you are purchasing superior oils is to go to a good herbalist or health food store, or contact the International Federation of Aromatherapists (see their address at the back of this book). Avoid stores that are oriented toward the cosmetic and beauty end of the market.

Be guided by price. The more expensive the oil, the more pure it is likely to be. Rose, for example, requires 5 tons of the flower to make just 1 kilogram (less than 2.2 pounds) of essential oil. Thus, if you are offered a "rose" oil at a price that seems reasonable, you can be almost sure that it has been adulterated in some way, perhaps by the addition of geraniol or citronellol.

Because the oils are susceptible to heat, light, and air, they must be kept in dark glass containers. You should endeavor to store them under similar conditions. Clear plastic bottles are definitely not recommended.

Aromatherapy is not merely about smelling nice and sweetly perfumed. It is a therapy and should be respected as such. Just as you would not expect your medical practitioner to prescribe medication that was substandard, so you should not be prepared to accept anything less than the best that is available, either when you make your own purchase or when you consult an aromatherapist.

5

Aromatherapy in Practice

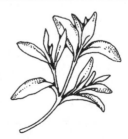

Having decided that you wish to take advantage of aromatherapy's many health and beauty benefits, whether at home or by consulting an aromatherapist, you need to know just how to select and use the essential oils.

To begin with, you need to be clear about what you are trying to achieve—whether it is to resolve a particular health condition or skin complaint, treat an emotional problem, or deal with a combination of factors. You should then consult the index of ailments in chapter 11 to discover which oils are recommended for which condition. Having discovered which oils are suitable for your needs you should then refer to the index of popular oils in chapter 10 to learn more about the one(s) you have selected. This will give you more information about the essence itself and how it works so that you can decide whether it really is the best for you.

If you can, smell the oil before you purchase or use it, particularly if you are trying to relieve an emotional problem. Some aromatherapists believe that if you dislike a particular aroma, no matter how "suitable" it appears to be on paper, you should not go ahead with it, and that if you are drawn to a smell, then it may be that the qualities that oil possesses are ones you actually need. Other aromatherapists would not agree. They believe that the chemical components of the aroma and how they work on the body are of primary importance.

WHAT NOTES ARE

Consideration should be given to the volatility or *note* of a particular oil. This is especially relevant if you want to blend oils. Most essential oils are classified as having top notes, middle notes, or base notes. The top notes are highly volatile. They act quickly, evaporate quickly, and stimulate the mind and body. They smell sharp. Middle notes are more stable. They last longer and are more involved in the physical functioning of the body, such as digestion. Base notes are the least volatile, and are often used to *fix* (hold on to) the more volatile oils and increase their staying power. Base notes have a relaxing, sedative effect, tend to blend in well with other aromas, and often smell sweeter and heavier than the other essences.

Examples of oils with top notes are cypress, lemon, peppermint, and tea tree. Some middle-note oils are chamomile, myrrh, ylang-ylang, pine, and rosemary. Base-note oils include sandalwood, patchouli, frankincense, and cedarwood.

When it comes to blending you will want to use the oils that are appropriate for your symptoms, as well as the cause of those symptoms. For example, if you are treating a headache you will see from the index of ailments that chamomile, lavender, peppermint, rosemary, and rose can all be used to treat this condition. If the headache is due to tension, you may want to add an oil that addresses that problem, too, such as marjoram or sandalwood.

You will find that the same oils can be used to treat a number of complaints and that different oils can be used to treat the same complaint. This is where it may help to use the notes as a guide, perhaps selecting a fast-acting top note for an immediate effect and combining it with a base note in order to prolong those effects and to relax you if that is also what you need.

There are a variety of ways in which the oils can be administered, which were mentioned briefly in earlier chapters. However, at the risk of repetition, they are massage, compresses and poultices, baths and saunas, inhalation, and mouthwashes. We will go into more detail about massage and bathing techniques in later chapters, here, we will begin our discussion of practice with massage oils.

CREATING YOUR OWN MASSAGE OILS

Custom-blending your own massage oils is one of the delights of practicing aromatherapy. (We describe massage techniques in chapter 9.)

First Conduct a Skin Test

If you are going to use essential oils in massage, you should do a skin test first, especially if you suffer from hay fever or some other allergy. *Always conduct such a test before using the oils on children and the elderly.* To conduct a skin test, apply one drop of oil with a cotton ball to the inside of the elbow, the back of the wrist, or under the arm. Leave unwashed for twenty-four hours. If the area erupts in a rash or itches, do not use that oil.

Carrier Oils

Essential oils should never be applied *neat* (undiluted) for massage. They should always be diluted in a carrier or base oil. A number of oils that are particularly suitable for mixing with essential oils also have properties which are beneficial to the individual (such as containing vitamins A, D, and E), particularly if they are cold-pressed. (Cold-pressing is a method of extracting oils without using heat or chemicals. Although cold-pressed oils can be more expensive, they retain more nutrients than oils expressed using other methods.) In addition, these carrier oils can help to balance and stabilize an essential oil. The vitamin E in wheatgerm oil, for example, acts as an antioxidant and enhances the keeping power of a massage oil once the essence has been blended with another vegetable oil. The usual life for a massage oil after dilution is only two months, but nearer three if wheatgerm oil is added.

The best carrier oils for essential oils are almond, grapeseed, soybean, wheatgerm, peach or apricot kernel, avocado, corn, sunflower, calendula, and castor. The oil should be able to penetrate the skin easily. It should also be 100 percent pure and unrefined. Some aromatherapists like to use a fragrant oil such as coconut, sesame, or olive oil. Others prefer to use an oil with little scent of its own, such as those listed in the first sentence of this paragraph.

The almond oil used in aromatherapy is extracted from the sweet almond (*Prunus amygdalus var. dulcis*). It has nourishing and revitalizing properties and is beneficial for dry and wrinkled hands, eczema, and skin irritations. Castor oil is more viscous and may have to be mixed with another oil to make it more penetrating, but it also has benefits for eczema and very dry skin. Grapeseed has a consistency almost like that of water and is therefore very easily absorbed. It is more astringent in its effects and thus is useful for such conditions as acne. Soybean oil is easily absorbed and is known to lower cholesterol levels in the bloodstream.

Wheatgerm oil, which is especially good for skin conditions because of its high content of vitamin E, is usually added to another base oil (just a drop or two) because it is quite rich and heavy. Avocado is another rich, heavy oil. An aromatherapist may well use a carrier oil that is a blend of oils such as wheatgerm, avocado, and grapeseed. Calendula oil, from a variety of marigold, helps to reduce inflammation and can be used for circulatory, digestive, menstrual, muscular, nervous, and skin disorders. It is often blended with other carrier oils because it is quite expensive.

Mineral oils have no value for aromatherapy because they are not able to penetrate the skin.

Quantities and Concentrations

Just as aromatherapy is a very individual therapy in terms of which essential oils to use, so the proportion of essential oil to carrier oil is also variable. However, more is not necessarily better—experience has shown that smaller amounts may achieve far more, particularly if the problem is an emotional or mental one. It is best, when starting with essential oils, to make up average concentrations. The more experience you gain, the more you will be able to experiment so as to obtain the maximum effect from your preparation.

To begin with, you may just want to make up enough of a massage oil for one session. It is helpful to acquire a 15-milliliter (equivalent to about 1 tablespoon) plastic measuring spoon for this purpose. The concentration of essential oil should be from ½ percent to no more than 3 percent of the carrier oil. The concentration will depend on the individual being massaged—his or her skin type and age—and the purpose for which the oil is being used as well as on the strength of the essential oil itself.

If you are going to apply the oil to the face, if the subject of the massage is a child or elderly, or if the skin is sensitive, you should start with a ½ percent concentration. If no irritation results after the initial application, then you can try increasing the concentration to 1 percent and then 2 percent. If an essential oil is very strong, it should not be used in concentrations above 1 to 1½ percent. (Please see the cautions section later in the chapter.)

To make up enough massage oil for one massage:

½ percent	3 drops essential oil to every 30 milliliters (2 tablespoons) carrier oil
1 percent	3 drops essential oil to every 15 milliliters (1 tablespoon) carrier oil
2 percent	6 drops essential oil to every 15 milliliters carrier oil
3 percent	9 drops essential oil to every 15 milliliters carrier oil

Use the 2 and 3 percent concentrations for body massage, subject to the cautions mentioned later.

You may want to make up larger amounts of facial or massage oils. These can then be stored in dark glass bottles for from two to three months. Fill a 50-milliliter (66-ounce) glass bottle with the carrier oil.

To make up 50 milliliters of massage oil:

½ percent	5 drops essential oil to 50 milliliters carrier oil
1 percent	10 drops essential oil to 50 milliliters carrier oil
2 percent	20 drops essential oil to 50 milliliters carrier oil
3 percent	30 drops essential oil to 50 milliliters carrier oil

If you want to use a blend of essential oils, you should make up the blend first and then add the suggested number of drops of the *combined* oils to the carrier. It is worth labeling the bottle containing the initial blend with types and proportions of the oils used.

COMPRESSES AND POULTICES

Bruises, sprains, pains, congestion, and skin irritations can be treated by using the age-old methods of compresses and poultices. In fact, the use of poultices was one of the first methods devised by humans for treating the sick.

Compresses

A compress may be hot or cold. If an injury is recent and there is bruising, swelling, and inflammation, or for a headache, a cold compress is advised. Hot compresses are better for old injuries, menstrual pain, cystitis, muscle pains, boils, and other skin conditions. For a compress, you need a soft piece of fabric—flannel, lint, towels, or old sheets are best. Lint should not be medicated. Sometimes cotton wool can be used (make sure it is real and not synthetic or a blend), although it has a tendency to absorb too much moisture.

If you are making a cold compress, put 6 to 10 drops of essential oil into half a liter (about 1 pint) of ice-cold water. Place the fabric on the top of the water and squeeze it to prevent it from dripping but not so much that it becomes dry. Put the compress on the area to be treated and wrap thin plastic around it. Secure it if necessary. The compress should remain in place until it has warmed up to body temperature, at which point it may need replacing.

For a hot compress, the quantities of water and essential oil are the same, but the water should be as hot as you can manage to bear. The compress should be renewed once it has cooled to body temperature. It sometimes helps to place a prewarmed towel over the compress, followed by a blanket. Ideally, compresses should be left in place for about two hours.

If you want to treat the back with a warm compress, you will need a larger piece of material. The water should then be placed in a bowl big enough to accommodate the size of the material. Add 10 drops of essential oil and allow the material to soak up the liquid. Place a warm towel on a bed, followed by plastic sheeting, and then by the compress. The person being treated should lie down on top of the compress and be covered by a warm blanket.

Poultices

Poultices consist of herbs that are applied, either raw or mashed, directly to the body. The herbs may be moistened first. Some poultices may be left exposed to the air; others might be wrapped in a cloth, which is then placed on the area needing attention. The most common poultices are linseed or mustard, which relieve chest complaints and skin problems.

The seeds of linseed are easily crushed. When liquid is added they swell in size and retain heat well. Use between 35 grams (1.5 ounces) and 100 grams (3.5 ounces), depending on the size of the area to be covered. The linseeds should be ground up using either a mortar and pestle or a food processor and then mixed with sufficient hot water to make a paste. You can then add 2 to 5 drops of essential oil. Spread the mixture on a piece of gauze or muslin, which should then be covered with a second piece of the material. Make sure that the ends of the material are folded over so that the contents do not fall out. Place the hot poultice on the affected area and leave until cool, about ten minutes. This preparation can be applied to the face, but as linseed is rather sticky, you will need to use a flower water to help remove it.

Mustard seed poultices should not be applied to the face. They are best used on the back and chest. Again, the seeds should be ground and boiling purified water should then be added to form a paste. You also could make a mustard poultice by adding mustard powder to a linseed or oatmeal paste. The poultice should be applied warm. You will find that the skin becomes hot and red. If left on for longer than ten minutes the skin begins to swell, so you should adhere strictly to times. After the poultice has been removed, make sure that you wash your hands. You will then need to apply a soothing agent, such as talcum powder or cornstarch, to the treated area.

A paste made from organic oats can be a good base for an essential oil poultice. Oatmeal is soothing to skin inflamed by poison oak or insect bites and contains vitamin E.

INHALATION

If you have ever steamed your face as a beauty measure or to relieve the symptoms of a cold, inhalation using essential oils will not seem at all strange to you.

A simple way of inhaling an oil is to apply it neat to a handkerchief or paper towel (about 5 to 10 drops) and then sniff. If you have a cold, then a piece of fabric with drops added can be placed on your pillow at night to help relieve congestion. Or sprinkle the drops on the pillowcase itself. Even more simple still is to put a drop of essential oil onto your hand, rub your hands to warm them up, and then cup your hands over your nose, allowing no gaps, and inhale deeply.

Using steam to help breathe in essential oils is particularly useful for colds, flu, and coughs. *(If you suffer from asthma do not try this method because it could bring on an attack.)* Assuming that the method does not pose a hazard for you, fill a bowl with half a liter (about 2 cups) of almost boiling water and add 2 to 4 drops of essential oil, depending on the strength of the oil. Breathe in the scented steam for between five and ten minutes. The treatment is rendered more effective if you keep your head and the bowl covered with a towel to make a sort of tent. You may need to repeat the treatment three times a day.

MOUTHWASH

To keep your mouth fresh and infection free, 2 drops of essential oils can be added to one cup of water. It is best to store this in a screw-top bottle, which can then be shaken each time it is used so that the oil is dispersed throughout. The best oils to use for fresh breath are mint and lemon. If you are treating a mouth infection or gum disorder, use tea tree oil. In all cases, distilled or springwater will provide the best results. Mouthwashes should *not* be swallowed.

INTERNAL USE

The internal use of essential oils is controversial. Some practitioners are very much against this practice. For the purpose of this book, internal use of essential oils, vinegars, and the herbs themselves is not recommended.

OTHER APPLICATIONS

Bathing is a well-recognized treatment to which we devote all of chapter 6. Using aromatherapy to keep the skin in good condition is discussed in chapter 8. Of course, you can always use essential oils just because you like the smell and want to perfume yourself and your environment.

To perfume a room, you can purchase essential oil burners and aromatherapy rings, which you impregnate with the oil and then place on your lightbulb so that the heat evaporates the oil and gives off the scent. A much cheaper and equally effective way of achieving the same result is to put 1 to 2 drops of oil onto a damp piece of cotton wool or fabric, which you then place on a radiator. Or try putting the drops onto a lightbulb while it is still cold. You can make an atomizer with a plastic spray bottle filled with water and a few drops of oil.

Spraying a room with essential oils is extremely beneficial if the occupant is sick. This practice helps to disinfect a room and thus prevent the spread of germs. Pine, eucalyptus, clove, cinnamon, rosemary, lavender, thyme, peppermint, lemon, and tea tree oils are especially useful.

Whether your aim is to create an atmosphere for a good night's sleep or for a party, be sure to choose the oils that will enhance that effect—chamomile, lavender, or clary sage for bedtime; bergamot, orange, or lemon to add zest to a gathering.

To perfume yourself, either for pleasure or to lift yourself up if you are feeling morose, you can use essential oils either singly or together. Frankincense, sandalwood, and/or lavender are excellent choices. Make up the blend by adding 2 to 3 drops of oil to 30 milliliters (2 tablespoons) of either water, wax, or an oil, depending on whether you want to make an aromatic water for splashing on after a shower or bath, or a skin perfume.

CAUTIONS

As we have mentioned, essential oils can be toxic and should be regarded with respect. As a rule, do *not* take the oils internally.

Sassafras should *never* be used in aromatherapy. Do not apply the following oils to the skin: cinnamon bark, cinnamon leaf, clove. If you are inexperienced, do not use pennyroyal, thuja, sage (clary sage, however, is safe), wintergreen, or thyme.

If you are sunbathing, you must avoid taking beforehand bergamot, lemon, orange, mandarin, grapefruit, lime, or verbena because they can cause the skin to pigment temporarily.

The fragrance industry has compiled a list of oils that should only be used in a restricted way. In aromatherapy the oils that fall within this restricted category include angelica, verbena, cassia, cinnamon, and cumin. Other oils that require close supervision are coriander and hyssop.

As for pregnancy, some aromatherapists maintain that no essential oils should be administered in any form, since some can have an adverse effect on the pregnancy. Other aromatherapists advocate their use because there can be benefits to the pregnant mother. If you are pregnant, consult an aromatherapist first before applying *any* oils. You also will want to refer to chapter 7, which discusses aromatherapy and pregnancy so that you are aware of the choices that can be made in conjunction with an aromatherapist.

It is possible to have an allergic reaction to an essential oil and you will recall the skin test that was mentioned earlier. If you have very sensitive skin, basil, bergamot, peppermint, lemongrass, ginger, ylang-ylang, verbena, and geranium oil may cause a reaction, especially if the dilutions are over $1\frac{1}{2}$ to 2 percent and if the area to which the oil is being applied is the face or a similar sensitive spot.

Finally, before using any oils, be sure to consult the index of oils (chapter 10), which contains the contraindications for each of those listed.

CONSULTING AN AROMATHERAPIST

Each aromatherapist has his or her own approach to the discipline, one which reflects his or her training, interests, and leanings. Some may, for example, include reflexology and shiatsu in the repertoire of skills they have to offer. Some are more clinical in their diagnosis and prescription of a suitable remedy. Others have a more spiritual bias. Or they may have trained in herbalism or nutrition. Whatever their style, all aromatherapists aim to treat the whole person and will devise a program to suit the individual's temperament, symptoms, and lifestyle.

It is very important that you find a therapist whom you can trust and open up to. Remember the mind/body connection and the importance of empathy in the process of healing. Because of this holistic approach, you can expect an initial consultation to last for some time—usually from an hour to an hour and a half. The aromatherapist will want to ask you questions about yourself, your way of looking at the world, your lifestyle, your pattern of illness/healing, any crises that you may have experienced, and your symptoms and how they manifest themselves. (You'll find the list of addresses at the back of this book helpful should you decide to contact a professional aromatherapist for a consultation.)

FREQUENTLY ASKED QUESTIONS ABOUT AROMATHERAPY

The following is an excerpt from a conversation with Nadine Artemis, a respected Canadian aromatherapist who owns and operates Osmosis: Everyday Aromatherapy, Canada's first full concept aromatherapy store.

Question   Where do you place aromatherapy in the field of healing?

Answer   As a complementary therapy that treats the mind, body, and emotions in a holistic manner.

Question   How do the aromatherapeutic techniques actually help?

Answer   Aromatherapy works on a number of levels to heal the body mentally, physically, and emotionally. When essential oils are inhaled, they work extremely fast, bypassing the blood-brain barrier and going directly to the hypothalamus where the essential oils release various neurochemicals. For example, lavender essential oil will release seratonin, which has a sedative, calming effect; therefore lavender is excellent for insomnia and migraines. Another example is jasmine, which releases endorphins that can create feelings of energy and euphoria.

When inhaled, essential oils also affect the limbic system (the oldest "reptilian" part of the brain). The limbic system governs memory, emotions, sexuality, and subjective feelings. Thus, aromatherapy can be very effective in dealing with times of transition, such as grief. Even if a person has no sense of smell (*anosmia*), aromatherapy can still be quite effective.

The term "aromatherapy" is slightly misleading, since this implies that its effects work only through the sense of smell. But the essential oils also affect the body on a physical level, when the tiny essential oils penetrate the skin and then enter the bloodstream and lymph systems, where they eliminate toxins, generate circulation, and calm inflammation. For example, the essential oil of rosemary stimulates mental activity and clarifies emotions, while on a physical level it helps generate circulation, aiding arthritis and varicose veins.

Question   Do the remedies that you've outlined get to the cause of the problem or is it more a case of alleviating the symptoms?

Answer   I think aromatherapy can be viewed as both a therapy for treating symptoms and a preventative aid. For example, essential oils can clear up some of the worst cases of eczema but the eczema will keep returning if the person has a food allergy and does not eliminate that item from his diet.

Many essential oils are wonderful immune stimulants and can keep the body in a healthy state. The massage used in aromatherapy contributes as well. I think that using the oils alone is not sufficient. For example, if you persist in drinking and smoking, using oils is not going to be that effective. It is important to engage the body and the mind.

Question   Can aromatherapy be used to treat all types of illnesses and conditions, or are there limitations?

Answer   This is a difficult question to answer because it varies not only from practitioner to practitioner but from country to country. In France, for example, doctors use aromatherapy for a variety of ailments, and even prescribe essential oils for internal use, in the same way as conventional doctors use drugs. In the United States and Canada, the majority of aromatherapists are not medically trained, so they tend to concentrate on aromatherapy as a means of reducing stress—which in itself can trigger a healing effect.

Question   Can anyone treat themselves using aromatherapy at home, even for quite serious illnesses?

Answer   I wouldn't say serious illnesses, no. You would need help from a holistic practitioner who would take an overall look at your illness and your whole lifestyle. Otherwise you are just treating the illness symptomatically, which never really does much. For instance, if you have athlete's foot, you can put lavender oil on it and it may go away. But, on the other hand, if you're not addressing the cause, which may be a symptom of stress, vitamin B deficiency, or something else, the athlete's foot may come back again. In other words, there may be a need for a deeper treatment.

Question   Is it wise to stick to one oil or opt for a combination in a treatment?

Answer   Using one essential oil can be very effective; however, when essential oils are combined, they create a synergistic effect, meaning the sum of the parts is greater than the whole. Therefore a blend of three to five essential oils has numerous properties that can treat numerous conditions. Because most symptoms do not exist in a vacuum there usually are a few to treat. In addition, many essential oils share similar properties and everyone has very individual, subjective responses, so what might clear up one person's asthma, may not clear up another's.

Question   Can orthodox medication for an ailment be used in conjunction with aromatherapy?

Answer   I wouldn't actually say to someone that you mustn't take this drug. Most of the clients I see don't take them, which is why they are trying alternative medicine. However, I think aromatherapy can be very effective treating some of side effects that are caused by conventional medicine. I wouldn't say that orthodox drugs counteract the essential oils, However, you must be careful mixing some essential oils with drugs because of the effects the two have on each other.

Question   Can aromatherapy be used safely in conjunction with other alternative therapies such as acupuncture, homeopathy, etc.?

Answer   With acupuncture, I don't think there is a problem, although this depends on the practitioner. Some acupuncturists would say that it's best if you just have one treatment at a time; otherwise you don't know if the treatment is working. If the acupuncturist agrees, I think that gentle massage with a very low dilution of oil would be harmonious, because it's all about balance.

Some homeopaths are strictly against using any aromatics—believing that even toothpaste will act as an antidote to some of the remedies—whereas others disagree. There isn't really any definitive answer but, traditionally, eucalyptus and peppermint and, perhaps, camphor, have been known to act as antidotes, as does coffee, simply because it is so aromatic. It's best to ask the homeopath.

Question   As a practicing aromatherapist, would you be happy for a patient to undergo homeopathic treatment or acupuncture at the same time as taking essential oils?

Answer   Yes, as long as not too many treatments are mixed at the same time. Massage, in general, is such a good relaxant that it enhances the internal conditions which help to trigger our immune defenses.

Question   Speaking of massage, it wasn't until this century that massage was introduced as part of aromatherapy treatment. How crucial is it to aromatherapy?

Answer   Before Marguerite Maury's use of massage in the 1950s, doctors tended to use essential oils as simply another form of herbal medicine to treat external conditions. In France, doctors still do not use massage very much. I think massage is perhaps the most important part of the therapy as a means of relieving stress. Most illness is the result of disharmony of the emotions and the mind and I think massage is important because it uses both the senses of touch and smell.

But the application of essential oils combined with carrier oils to the body (without massage) and inhalation of essential oils can also be effective. This makes aromatherapy a practical, accessible, empowering way for people to maintain their health on an everyday basis

Question   These days essential oils are commonly available. Are there any guidelines to purchasing oils?

Answer   Essential oils are obtainable, but pure essential oils are not always commonly available. The quality of essential oils varies depending on country of origin, method of distillation, and soil and climate conditions. It is *very* important to buy essential oils that have the Latin binomial on the label. The Latin name is important because chamomile, for instance, could be Roman (*Anthemis nobilis*) or German (*Matricaria chamomilla*), each of which contains very different properties. "Blue chamomile" is often sold with *tanacteum annum* inside, not the true *Matricaria*, which is more expensive.

It is also important to know what part of the plant was used—the leaf or the bark (cinnamon), the needles or the branches (juniper)—because they will have very different properties and one part of the plant may not be as safe or desirable as the other. Read the labels, follow your nose! My advice would be to smell many different types of oils (even synthetic) because then your nose can begin to decipher quality and differences between the oils. An oil can also be checked by dropping it on a piece of paper; if it does not evaporate, then it probably has been diluted in a carrier oil.

Question   How do the essential oils boost the immune system?

Answer   They release endorphins (brain hormones) that make us feel happy and when we are happy we are less likely to become ill. Thyme, chamomile, and lavender are widely used in France to boost white cell production. Aromatherapy is a multifaceted therapy that works on many levels. Essential oils also work on and stimulate the glandular system as well as working with the lymph system to eliminate toxins.

Question   Are there any conditions that must not be treated with essential oils—for example, asthma or serious heart conditions?

Answer   Provided there are no allergies, most oils are safe. I would give the patient oils to smell and see if the reaction is favorable or not. Asthmatics must avoid steam inhalation—not because of the oils, but the steam itself. But this is very individual; some asthmatics can tolerate many oils while others cannot. Furthermore, some essential oils are not recommended for pregnancy or epilepsy and some are phototoxic.

Question   Please give an example of a strong oil.

Answer   Ginger is a strong oil, a rubefacient. It causes redness in the skin, which is part of its healing properties, bringing warmth into the area. But, to some people, that redness may flare up into a rash if you use it in a very high concentration. Never use ginger oil neat. Dilutions should vary according to the strength of the oil. The maximum concentration of ginger would be only 1 drop in 15 milliliters (about 1 tablespoon) of oil, whereas lavender could be as concentrated as 9 drops per 15 milliliters. No oil is the same.

Question   How much experience is necessary to use essential oils?

Answer   If you have no experience, keep to very low concentrations and avoid the known potentially risky oils. Clove oil is one that should never be used directly on the skin, for example. It's a matter of being sensible.

Question   How long does it take to train as an aromatherapist?

Answer   Qualifications in anatomy and physiology are necessary and a good course will last at least a year. But, at the moment, the laws in the United States and Canada do not demand any qualifications before a person sets up as a practicing aromatherapist. Some people just attend a weekend course and set up in practice, although they would not be on the list of an accredited register of aromatherapists. I would be sure to check the credentials of any aromatherapist carefully before a consultation.

Question   Do you find that people come to you as a last resort?

Answer   Some people turn to aromatherapy as a last resort but it is usually because they were not aware of various complementary medicines. Many people discover aromatherapy for different reasons, whether it be for therapy, a way for them to make their office smell stimulating, or as a natural alternative to synthetic perfume.

Question   On average, how many sessions would it take for a course of treatment?

Answer   Usually, about half a dozen. Massage is ongoing; some people need more sessions depending on their lifestyle and stress levels.

Question   Where should one look for a practitioner?

Answer   The best thing to do is to contact an accredited association in your country for a list of reputable aromatherapists. [See the list of addresses at the end of this book for professional organizations to contact.] Apart from that, it's word of mouth. You can't only go with qualifications. You have to get along well with your aromatherapist. It doesn't matter how good the aromatherapist is if your personalities clash.

Question   What would you say is the most important healing aspect of aromatherapy?

Answer   In addition to the tender loving care that an aromatherapist provides, I would say that the most important healing aspect is the main tool of aromatherapy—the essential oils! Without them aromatherapy as we know it would not exist.

6

Aromatherapy
and Water

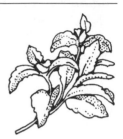

Along with herbal remedies, the use of water to treat the many and varied complaints that assail us is one of the oldest therapies known to humankind. Its history parallels that of herbal medicine and aromatherapy. The main developers of *hydrotherapy* (water healing) were the Egyptians—the same civilization that turned the use of aromatic substances into both an art and a science.

A Brief History of Bathing and Western Civilization

The ancient Egyptians attached special importance to bathing, turning this pleasurable pastime into a therapy by combining aromatic substances and water to effect a cure. Wealthy women often spent much of the day bathing—starting with a cold bath, followed by a tepid one, and then, finally, a hot bath, which was followed by a massage with one of the more sought after essential oils, such as cypress or cedarwood.

Although the Greeks adopted many of the Egyptians' bathing practices, bathing didn't catch on to the same degree. The Greek physician Hippocrates prescribed bathing and springwater to treat his patients, but in general it was the Greek men who adopted the practice, using the public marble baths, while the women more discreetly tended to their hygiene in the privacy of their own homes.

No one who has visited the historic city of Bath in England or the city of Rome can be in any doubt about the importance that the Roman civilization attached to water. Again, public bathing was a mostly male occupation but its prominence in society was far greater than in Greece. The public baths, or *thermae*, were often housed in magnificent buildings, especially those frequented by the emperors, who built the most luxurious of them. Of particular merit are the baths built by the emperor Caracalla in the third century B.C.; there were more than a thousand public baths in Rome itself at that time.

With the expansion of the Roman Empire throughout Europe, the popularity of bathing spread, then declined with the collapse of the empire. Interest in bathing was revived briefly in the thirteenth century by the Crusaders returning from the East, where bathing was quite popular.

In the sixteenth century, water began to assume greater importance in Europe with the development of water "cures" at the sites of mineral springs and wells, with doctors prescribing strict programs of drinking and bathing. New techniques were introduced. Steam baths, for example, became popular with the Turks and, later, the French for the purposes of relaxation and treatment. By the seventeenth century, the public was much more disposed to bathing, and bathing became more and more a part of daily life. In England steam baths started to become popular.

Over the next two hundred years, hydrotherapy increased its influence and the number of different water treatments grew. Many towns and cities around Europe became famous for their spas, and wealthy households would often do a tour of these centers, particularly if they had a sickly member of the family. The sorts of treatments that were offered included full baths, hip baths, hand and foot baths, steam baths, compresses, and water dressings.

With the diversification of water treatments came the introduction of special concoctions to increase the efficacy of the treatments—plant substances and essential oils in particular. The two practitioners who had the most influence in the development of medicinal baths were Vincent Priessnitz, who used only pure cold water treatments, and Pastor Kneecap, who made great use of medicinal plants in his hot and cold water treatments. It was largely as a result of Pastor Kneecap's efforts that essential oils became common in hydrotherapy.

BALNEOTHERAPY

In modern times, baths using herbs or essential oils have come to be known as *balneotherapy* and it is possible for many of us to give ourselves a treatment in our own homes. In fact, you could spend the whole weekend having a course of treatment without the inconvenience of traveling to a therapy center. You could choose individual oils to suit your own requirements or obtain essences that have been especially developed for use in balneotherapy. Of course, if you are treating a particular health condition, you should always consult a qualified aromatherapist first.

Therapeutic baths are especially helpful for colds, rheumatism, and, of course, relaxation. Remember that the skin, far from being an impermeable barrier, actually allows very small molecules to pass through it. It has been found that during a one-hour bath, provided the body is totally immersed, 16 to 20 milliliters of pure water can permeate the outer layer (epidermis) of the skin. The molecules of essential oils are much smaller than those of water and, for that reason, are absorbed 100 times better than water. Recall that once absorption of essential oils has taken place, they are then circulated in the bloodstream so that they act at a very basic level in the body. Pine baths, for example, have been shown to increase white blood cell counts, thus enhancing the immune function.

Research shows that essential oils act on two levels—the local and the general. The local effects are produced by the warming effects of the oils. Once the oils have permeated the skin, they stimulate the circulation of the blood, which, in turn, produces a rise in skin temperature. More general long-term benefits include continued stimulation of the blood circulation and enhanced metabolic processes and, of course, warmth is associated with reduction in pain. This last is of particular interest to those people who suffer from diseases of the locomotor system and from chronic inflammation. Rheumatism, neuralgia, myalgia, strains, contusions, and sports injuries may all be successfully treated by essential oils added to water.

Aromatic oils added to baths also work through inhalation, through breathing in the aromatic molecules, which are then absorbed into the bloodstream from the lungs, and also through the actual smell, which is transmitted to the brain through the olfactory nerves, thereby producing a mental and emotional response.

METHODS OF BATHING

You will by now have gathered that bathing can be more than just having a bath. In fact, balneotherapy involves a number of techniques depending on the desired result. If the whole body requires treatment then full baths and showers are recommended, although the latter are not so useful if aromatic substances are to be employed. Sitz baths are especially devised for accommodating the bottom, hips, and lower abdomen and are prescribed for conditions that relate only to those areas, such as gynecological ailments. You can improvise at home by using a bowl or baby bathtub. Hot-and-cold baths (also known as hand or foot baths) are useful when it is not practical or feasible to take a full bath.

Standard Baths

If you are going to have a full bath, then you should ensure that it is deep enough for your shoulders to be immersed. You must also keep to the following temperature requirements. The temperature of a hot bath should be no greater than 99 to 108 degrees F (37 to 42° C). Twenty minutes is the maximum safe duration of a hot bath. Any longer and you might feel dizzy or light-headed when you get out. The temperature for a tepid bath ranges from 92 to 97 degrees F (33 to 36° C) and you can remain in it for up to an hour. Needless to say, a cold bath is only of a short duration, with the temperature between 59 and 68 degrees F (15 to 20° C). Afterwards rub yourself briskly with a towel.

Sitz Baths

For a hot sitz bath, the temperature should range from 99 to 108 degrees F (37 to 42° C). Immerse your hips and bottom so that the water comes up to your waist. Begin with a two-minute bath on the first day and increase the time gradually over the next few days so that eventually you reach a maximum of ten minutes.

For a cold sitz bath, the temperature should be from 59 to 68 degrees F (15 to 20° C). The procedure is the same as for hot sitz baths.

To take a hot-and-cold sitz bath in one session, you will need two large basins, one containing hot water and the other cold. First, sit in the hot water while your feet are soaking in the cold water for approximately three minutes. Next, sit in the cold basin with your feet in the hot water for one minute, then revert to the previous arrangement. Repeat the procedure two or three times.

Hot-and-Cold Baths

These are also known as hand or foot baths. "Hot" means as hot as you can bear and "cold" as cold as you can bear (using ice if necessary). If you are bathing your hands, find two bowls—one for the hot water, one for the cold—large enough to allow you to place both hands and wrists under water. For a foot bath, you will need two bowls deep enough to cover your feet and ankles.

Start with the hot water for one minute, then cold for twenty seconds; continue switching from hot to cold for about ten minutes. You should finish with a quick cold bath.

Using Essential Oils in the Bath

In Germany, the use of essential oils with bathing has been developed to a high degree and it is possible to buy mixtures prepared specifically for these purposes. In one, turpentine oil, camphor oil, rosemary oil, and eucalyptus oil have been mixed to produce a cold water bath product designed to treat respiratory problems. Essential oil products for adding to hot baths also can be obtained for treating rheumatism or for relaxation. The oils are chosen for their warming properties and for stimulating blood circulation. Each of the oils complements the actions of the others so that a complete treatment is afforded.

To obtain such products, inquire first at a good health food store or herbalist. Suppliers often advertise in the classified section of alternative health magazines. But you can achieve much the same effects by following the recommendations in the index of oils in chapter 10 of this book. And by using the index, you can make up the blend of oils you feel are particularly appropriate for you.

THE BEST HERBS FOR BATHING PURPOSES

Many products on the market smell attractive, such as bath salts, and, no doubt, they do help to make bathing more enjoyable and relaxing. But they do not have any curative properties; they belong to the realm of cosmetics. Aromatherapy is concerned with more than just smelling nice, however, and the therapeutic aspects of aromatic oils are important. These can be mediated through pure bath oils that contain the *essences* (active principles) of the plant.

These essences could take the form of whole plant extracts, which tend to be syrupy in consistency, or the chopped-up plant itself, which is either placed in a bag put into the bathwater, or is used by way of a decoction. Or, of course, the essential oils could be added to the bathwater. The plants (or parts of plants) that have been found to have the best medicinal properties for bathing purposes are: pine, oak bark, valerian, melissa, rosemary, thyme, chamomile, yarrow, and lavender.

Pine

The Norwegian spruce is the most commonly used pine, followed by the silver fir and the Scots pine. The greatest concentration of active principles is found in the young shoots of trees that are between sixty and eighty years old. Three types of extract are derived from these trees—pine needle, tannin (from the bark), and pine wood. Pine needle extract contains essential oil and 15 to 16 percent tannic acid. In tannin extract the tannin content is between 26 and 28 percent, which means that it has a greater capacity to irritate and is therefore mainly used to treat rheumatic conditions. Pine wood extract's essential oil content is much lower.

The extracts are obtained through a three-stage process. First, the essential oil is distilled from the plant material. Then the water-soluble parts are extracted. These are turned into a concentrated syrup and the essential oil is added back. It is important to ensure that the preparation you purchase is not a by-product of the paper industry if you want to use the extract for therapeutic purposes. Check the source with your supplier if you can. Of course, you can just use the essential oil but it will not contain tannin, an ingredient which is itself desirable. High-quality pine bath oils are commonly available in Europe. In the United States, try health food stores, which are more likely to carry quality products.

Pine baths are helpful for nervous diseases, rheumatism, and neuralgic conditions. A pine bath is simple to prepare, but you should obtain professional advice as to the temperature of the water and the length of time the bath should take. You also need to ensure that you rest for a sufficiently long period after the bath, which will depend on the purpose of the bath and the condition being treated. A resting time of at least half an hour is desirable, preferably an hour.

Oak Bark

Oak bark, from either the English oak or the durmast oak, is used particularly to treat chronic skin conditions and sweaty feet. Compresses have beneficial effects for weeping eczema and eye problems. However, unlike pine extract, oak bark does not contain any essential oil and is much higher in tannin (26 to 30 percent), which is why it is so effective for these ailments.

Its use differs, too, in that full baths of the bark are rare. Instead the plant substances are added to partial baths and compresses. A decoction can be made by adding a small handful of bark to a liter (about 1 quart) of water. The mixture is then boiled until it is reduced by half and the decoction is added to either a hand or a foot bath. If the bark is to be used in a compress, it is boiled for ten to fifteen minutes and then strained and used. It is possible to purchase good quality oak bark extract and the ideal dose for a partial bath is 5 to 15 milliliters (one teaspoon to one tablespoon) extract in a large bowl of hand-hot water.

Valerian

If you need to relax and particularly if you want a good night's sleep, then try adding 5 drops of the essential oil to a full bath.

Melissa

This plant also has sedative and relaxing properties and is of particular benefit for people who suffer from nervous heart conditions, insomnia, and restlessness. Whole plant extracts are usually recommended but good effects can be obtained by adding 5 to 10 drops of essential oil to a full tub of water.

Rosemary

Because rosemary is a stimulating plant, a rosemary bath should be taken in the morning, followed by rest. The plant contains camphor and acts on the circulatory and nervous systems. Hypotension, disorders of the veins, rheumatic pain, contusions, and sprains can all be helped. You could make an infusion of 50 grams of rosemary leaves (about 1¾ ounces) and half a liter of water (about 2 cups) to add to the bath. Alternatively, use 5 drops of the essential oil in a full tub of water.

Thyme

Thyme oil acts particularly through absorption and inhalation of the steam from hot water. It can help to calm coughs, including whooping cough, and is of benefit even for emphysema. Use no more than 5 drops in a full bath or 5 milliliters (1 teaspoon) of a blend.

Chamomile

Rather than being used for full baths, chamomile tends to be added to partial baths or compresses. Add 2 to 3 drops of the essential oil to a large bowl of hand-hot water. Chamomile helps wounds to heal, soothes skin irritations, such as eczema, and can relieve hemorrhoids.

Lavender

Like rosemary, lavender is a stimulant and a tonic for the nervous system. Again, the benefits of such a bath are mediated through absorption and the olfactory nerves in the nose and brain. Add 5 to 10 drops of the essential oil to a full tub of water.

7

Pregnancy and
Aromatic Oils

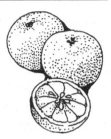

For most of us, the birth of a baby is a welcome event—something we may have planned and thought about with great care. For others, pregnancy may have come as a shock—perhaps the timing was bad. But whatever the circumstances, taking care of your own needs and finding the time to relax and pamper yourself through the use of aromatic oils is a very good way of helping you to adjust (and, perhaps, reconcile yourself) to the changes that are taking place within your body and the family unit.

In an ideal world, all pregnancies would be planned and each of us would have taken steps to bring our bodies to the state of optimum health prior to conception. This is important not only for the ease of pregnancy, but to strengthen sperm, eggs, and the conditions in which the unborn baby will grow. If you are fortunate enough to be planning on getting pregnant, you will be glad to learn that essential oils can benefit you even now.

Indeed, you can take a number of measures to ensure the best start to your pregnancy, and this is not just the woman's responsibility. Both partners need to look at their lifestyles. How much alcohol do you drink? Do you smoke? How much fresh fruit and vegetables do you consume? Do you have endless cups of coffee or tea? How stressed are you?

Excessive alcohol consumption in women can create toxic conditions that are potentially harmful to the developing embryo. In men, the result of excess alcohol may be infertility or damaged sperm. Insufficient consumption of fresh fruits and vegetables in both men and women can have similar consequences. Women with a folic acid deficiency (folic acid is found principally in dark green leafy vegetables) may bear a child with neural tube defect such as spina bifida. Vitamin C deficiency has been linked with poor quality sperm and a low sperm count. Smoking is known to adversely affect the birthweight of babies, who tend to be smaller and more prone to respiratory diseases. Too much tea can give rise to a zinc deficiency in the mother, which has also been linked to some birth defects.

Your aim should be to reduce or eliminate alcohol, tea, and coffee consumption; to give up smoking; and to eat a diet of fresh, whole foods that contains plenty of fruits, vegetables, complex carbohydrates such as whole grains, beans, pulses, and good quality protein—either from lean meat, chicken, and fish, or, if you are vegetarian, from well-combined vegetables, pulses (soybeans are a source of complete proteins), and whole grains. Eating well doesn't have to be boring. There are many books on the market with recipes designed to fit your lifestyle and budget.

If you are discontinuing use of birth control pills in order to conceive, it is advisable to wait at least three months before becoming pregnant. This is because the contraceptive interferes with folic acid levels in the body, which, as we discussed above, increases the risk of producing a baby with a birth defect. It is also better if the hormonal imbalances that can occur with the pill have a chance to normalize before pregnancy. If you have been using an intrauterine device as a contraceptive, it is worth checking to see that you do not have a pelvic infection which has gone undetected. Such an infection may affect your chances of conceiving.

USING ESSENTIAL OILS TO IMPROVE FERTILITY

Certain essential oils contain properties that are of particular benefit for those who are hoping to conceive. Many of these oils are found in the reproductive parts of plants—for example, the flowers, the aromas of which are designed to attract pollinating insects so that fertilization can take place. Essential oils from flowers, therefore, often contain alluring, aphrodisiac qualities, which not only help to create the right atmosphere, but actually can affect our reproductive organs and the balance of our hormones.

One flower that is especially associated with romance and feminine qualities is the rose. Hippocrates himself recommended the use of rose in obstetrics. At least three months before you expect to conceive, start to use rose essential oil from the *Rosa damascena* (or *rose otto*). This oil is believed to promote fertility and is effective for both partners. If the man wishes to increase his sperm count, he would find it beneficial to take warm baths containing 4 to 10 drops of the essential oil, taking care not to have hot baths as they can actually damage sperm. For the woman, rose can help to regulate the menstrual cycle and to tone the uterus. For best effect, take a sitz bath of tepid water with 3 to 7 drops of the oil. You will recall that such baths can easily be constructed by using a baby bathtub or bowl. (See chapter 6 for additional information on therapeutic baths).

In addition to these physical benefits, rose essential oil is a great relaxant, and what could be better for the prospective parents than to create a loving environment through massage? Try 4 to 7 drops of essential oil to 30 milliliters (2 tablespoons) of carrier oil.

Other essential oils are useful. *Pelargonium odorantissium* (or geranium, as it is commonly known) acts on the female reproductive organs in a similar way to rose—affecting the menstrual cycle and balancing the hormones. If relaxation is what is particularly needed, then bergamot (*Citrus aurantium bergamia*), neroli (*Citrus aurantium* var. amara), ylang-ylang (*Cananga odorata*), and clary sage (*Salvia sclarea*) can all help. A combination of some or all of these, plus rose, can be of particular benefit to a woman hoping to become pregnant. To 60 milliliters (4 tablespoons) of carrier oil, add 3 drops of rose, 4 drops of geranium, 3 drops of clary sage, 2 drops of ylang-ylang, and 2 drops of bergamot.

Use this mixture each night before falling asleep, applying it with the following massage technique. The entire abdomen should be massaged, starting at the inner rim of one of the pelvic bones, going along over the diaphragm and over the solar plexus (the pit of the stomach). After having gone around in a circle, focus on the area of the uterus. Hand movements should be small and circular, moving clockwise.

USING ESSENTIAL OILS AFTER CONCEPTION

Aromatherapists and others who work with essential oils are divided in their opinion as to whether essential oils should be used during pregnancy. The arguments against it are: the skin becomes more sensitive during pregnancy and it is not possible to predict how it will react to a particular oil; smells that were previously acceptable may now be perceived as unpleasant and may even cause nausea; and, most importantly, some essential oils are positively dangerous because they contain chemicals such as apiol and myristicine that can have an abortive effect or an adverse effect on the uterus.

Many practitioners who believe that a pregnant woman should avoid using essential oils suggest drinking herbal teas and using plants for infusions and in cooking instead.

Other therapists, while acknowledging the dangers of some essential oils and stressing the importance of avoiding these, believe that aromatic substances have much to offer throughout pregnancy and during birth. Even those therapists who express great concern about essential oils in pregnancy accept that some are so gentle they can be used with little harm. Lavender is one such oil. Much also depends on how the essential oil is administered. While direct contact with the skin may be inadvisable for certain oils, inhalation by means of a few drops in a bowl of warm water may be acceptable and even beneficial. The general view is that it is safe to use certain essential oils, but you must be especially conscientious about finding out which they are. If in doubt, do not use an oil, or consult a reputable aromatherapist first.

Women experience a variety of uncomfortable symptoms during pregnancy. Some of these can be attributed to the physical changes that occur in the body and others to lifestyle—perhaps you are trying to do your job without concession to your condition, or have older children who demand more of you than is physically possible. Changes can be made, however, to diet and daily regimes. Ask for extra help in taking children to school or their other activities. Eat smaller, more frequent meals; take vitamin and mineral supplements, if necessary. Be sure to get sufficient rest. You may find that essential oils make the adjustments easier and the symptoms more bearable.

Morning Sickness and Vomiting

Some women experience these symptoms right from the start of their pregnancy, but they are more commonly felt during the third month, when the placenta establishes itself. It is thought, too, that morning sickness may be the result of low blood sugar in the morning, or a deficiency of vitamin B_6. Some suggestions for alleviating the discomfort include having a snack of proteins, carbohydrates, and fruit before retiring to bed, and the same before getting up in the morning; keeping a supply of dry crackers with you to nibble on during the day; taking brewer's yeast or a yeast extract; and drinking sparkling mineral water. Some herbal teas can also be helpful, especially ginger, chamomile, lemon balm, meadowsweet, gentian, black horehound, and slippery elm.

Just having a pleasant and relaxing aroma around may be sufficient to provide relief. The easiest way of maintaining this is either to use an aromatic diffuser or to add a few drops of essential oil to a container of warm water so that the oil evaporates into the room. (A diffuser is more effective, however.) A good mix of oils is 3 drops of lavender (*Lavandula officinalis* or *Lavandula vera*) to 1 drop of peppermint (*Mentha pipperita*), plus 1 drop of another oil such as eucalyptus (*Eucalyptus globulus*) if other members of the family are suffering from colds or flu.

You can also use lavender oil in a cool compress applied to the forehead and in a warm compress on your chest. Peppermint oil sniffed from the bottle has also been found to be effective against nausea. As an aid against nausea when you go out of the house, place a drop of either lavender or peppermint oil onto a cotton handkerchief and keep it in a plastic bag in case you meet any smells that make you nauseous or give you a headache. Just breathe in deeply from the handkerchief as often as needed.

Peppermint and lavender also provide relief from headaches. Applying a drop of undiluted lavender oil to each temple has been found to work, as has the application of a cool peppermint oil compress to the forehead.

If you find that you are vomiting, try adding 7 drops of lemon (*Citrus limon*) or lavender oil to 30 milliliters (2 tablespoons) of carrier oil, which should then be massaged over the abdomen. Or you can smell this mixture. Remember, if your vomiting is severe, you must seek medical attention.

Painful Legs and Veins

Many women experience leg cramps, edema (excess water retention), varicose veins, and hemorrhoids during pregnancy. These are produced by the increase in the volume of blood in the body and the hormone progesterone, which softens the walls of the veins. Other factors may predispose a woman to these discomforts, such as weight gain or an insufficiency of vitamins B_6 and E.

If varicose veins do develop, the essential oils to try are cypress, geranium, lemon, and lavender. Apply them singly or as a blend in alternating warm and cool compresses to the affected area, keeping your legs raised. Disperse 1 to 2 drops of the essential oil into a bowl of water and gently lay the compress cloth on the surface of the water to attract the film. Bathing may also help. Just add 3 drops of cypress oil and 3 drops of lemon to a warm bath. Gentle massage, too, can help. To 60 milliliters (4 tablespoons) of carrier oil, add 7 drops of cypress oil and 7 drops of lemon. Start your massage by using gentle strokes, moving upward from the feet.

Hemorrhoids are a condition similar to varicose veins. Straining to pass a stool can also bring them on. Eating plenty of fruits, vegetables, and whole grains to ensure roughage in your diet will prevent any problems of elimination. Sitz baths are particularly beneficial if hemorrhoids do develop. Try a cool bath with 7 drops of lemon oil followed by a massage using the same mixture of lemon, cypress, and carrier oil as for varicose veins above.

If you suffer from swollen ankles or legs (edema), lavender, geranium, and rosemary (*Rosmarinus officinalis*) oils all can help, by encouraging drainage of excess fluid. A blend of the three oils (2 drops each) in 15 milliliters (1 tablespoon) of carrier oil can be massaged gently, using upward strokes, into the feet and ankles. Tepid to cool foot baths, to which are added 3 drops of geranium or lemon and 3 drops of lavender, can relieve the symptoms of hot, tired, or swollen feet. Full baths of lemon, mandarin (*Citrus reticulata*), or other citrus oils can act as a diuretic. Add 2 to 3 drops of essential oil to a full tub of water.

Stretch Marks

Whether or not you develop stretch marks will depend to some extent on your skin type. Dry, fair skin is more prone. However, you can take some steps to reduce the likelihood of them happening to you. A diet rich in cold-pressed vegetable oils (such as olive oil or sesame oil), which are high in vitamin E, will encourage greater elasticity of the skin. Vitamin C is particularly important for maintaining the structure of the skin.

Massage with vegetable oils is another way of deterring stretch marks. Wheatgerm, avocado, marigold, hazelnut, almond, and safflower oils can all be used separately or together, either in their own right or as a carrier for essential oils. Lavender, geranium, or mandarin are good aromas to add to the carrier. One good recipe for an anti-stretch-mark blend is 30 milliliters of hazelnut oil, 30 milliliters (2 tablespoons) of wheatgerm oil, 4 drops of neroli oil, 2 drops of carrot seed oil (*Daucus carota*), and 2 drops geranium oil. Massage with this mixture twice daily on the areas prone to stretch marks. You also could add the blend to a warm bath, adding seaweed extract or seawater concentrate. After patting yourself dry, smooth in more of the essential oil blend.

Other Skin Conditions

Acne and chloasma (a brownish pigmentation, often on the face) may arise during pregnancy. If you find yourself suffering from acne, undiluted lavender oil dabbed on in tiny amounts can help as can tea tree oil (*Melaleuca alternifolia*). Use just one drop of the oil.

For chloasma, a blend of 3 drops of lemon oil and 4 drops of myrtle (*Myrtus communis*) to 30 milliliters (2 tablespoons) of carrier oil, worked into the skin with cool water or a floral water, may do the trick.

Toning the Perineum

Apart from treating particular complaints, essential oils can be used to prepare for the birth itself. You can help to keep yourself relaxed and comfortable throughout the pregnancy through massage, either by yourself or with the assistance of your partner.

One particular area of the body deserves attention during pregnancy because it will be stretched to the utmost when the baby is born. It is, of course, the perineum, the skin between the vagina and the anus. When the baby is delivered this sometimes tears, or an episiotomy is performed by the midwife or doctor to make it easier for the baby to emerge. However, both tearing and episiotomies can be avoided through massage of the area with essential oils. A blend of 3 drops of lavender, 1 drop of geranium, and 30 milliliters (2 tablespoons) of wheatgerm oil makes a good massage oil. A qualified aromatherapist should be consulted to advise on the correct massage technique.

CHILDBIRTH

Research shows that fetal distress during labor can be considerably reduced through essential oil body massage (Kafan 1992). For the baby's benefit, as well as your own, you may want to make essential oils an integral part of the care you receive during labor. It is important to talk this over with your midwife or doctor beforehand, as well as talking with the person (your friend or partner) who will be supporting you. This will ensure that your wishes are known and respected by all involved, so that you can get on with the most important task of giving birth without distraction or resistance.

Your birthing kit may include blended oils for massage, which you should have made up at least three weeks before the due date (don't forget to store them in dark glass bottles); a selection of undiluted essential oils, which you can add to baths or use for compresses or inhalations; an aromatic diffuser; a plastic baby bathtub for sitz baths; and flannels and bowls for compresses.

Atmosphere is important. Essential oils that can promote a relaxing environment may be neroli, bergamot, rose, and frankincense. Use these in a diffuser or add 3 to 4 drops to a bowl of warm water. Lavender oil also is relaxing. When your cervix has dilated to 2 centimeters, a lavender bath will facilitate progress. If you want to be massaged between contractions, try using a blend of 20 drops of lavender oil and 8 drops of clary sage to 120 milliliters of carrier oil.

Where contractions need to be stimulated, try a jasmine (*Jasminum grandiflorum*) compress on your lower abdomen or sacrum. Or apply a compress of spikenard (*Nardostachys jatamansi*) if the pain is making you resist your contractions. Mix 8 drops of spikenard oil with 7 drops of jasmine and

---

Cautions

As has been stressed throughout this book, you must take great care in selecting your essential oils. They must be pure and extracted for therapeutic use. You must also ensure that you purchase the right species of plant because certain properties are often peculiar to that species only.

You should avoid the following completely while pregnant: ajowan, aniseed, basil, bitter almond, boldo, buchu, camphor, cornmint, cotton lavender, dove, fennel, horseradish, hyssop, *Lavandula stoechas*, mugwort, mustard, myrrh, oregano, parsley seed, pennyroyal, *Pimenta racemosa*, plecanthrus, rue, sage (clary sage is safe), sassafras, savin, savory, sweet birch, sweet marjoram, tansy, tarragon, thuja, thyme, wintergreen, wormseed, and wormwood.

---

3 drops of verbena and add to 120 milliliters of carrier oil. You can also use this for an abdominal massage.

If you are flagging, try a cool compress on your forehead. A sniff of lavender or peppermint can help if you suddenly feel nauseous.

AFTER THE BIRTH

After the birth, you may wish to relax in a warm aromatic bath. If your perineum has torn, you can help the healing process by taking baths to which you've added to 3 to 5 drops of lavender and myrrh essential oils. You could also massage the area with wheatgerm oil mixed with a few drops of lavender essential oil.

Babies can be a lot of work, and it takes time to adjust to the newest member of the family. This is where the restorative and relaxing properties of aromatic oils come into their own. Scent your home with those that you find particularly soothing, rest as much as you can, and remember, if you are having a particularly fraught day, it will pass.

8

Skin Care

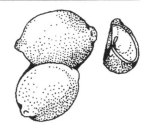

Few of us are blessed with perfect skin. Even those people who seem to go through life with a dewy complexion succumb from time to time to the occasional blemish or dry patch. When you consider what the skin has to put up with, both from the outside and from within, it is not surprising that imperfection is the norm. The saying about beauty being only skin deep implies superficiality but there is nothing superficial about the skin. It is a complex, layered structure that performs many different functions.

THE STRUCTURE OF SKIN

Skin has been described as the largest organ of our body. The bit that we see, and what we tend to think of as the skin, is called the *epidermis*. Even that, however, is made up of several layers of skin cells. The actual surface is composed of dead cells, which have traveled to the top in order to be shed to make way for new ones. The new cells are manufactured at the basal layer and move outwards toward the surface. As they do so, they lose their moisture and become flatter in the process. By the time they reach the topmost layer they have become brittle and flaky, which is not surprising when you consider that by that time they are composed primarily of keratin, the protein which makes up our nails and hair. As we age, the process of elimination and regeneration of cells slows down, which means that the skin surface is covered with a greater number of dead cells and it takes longer to replace them.

Below the epidermis is the *dermis*. This layer is very much alive. It is nourished by a myriad of small blood vessels, which also remove waste from the cells. Nerve endings are located in the dermis. These send messages about touch, pain, and temperature from the skin to the brain. Then there are the oil (sebaceous) and sweat glands.

The sebaceous glands open out onto the epidermis and are better known as pores. The purpose of the oil (sebum) is to keep the skin pliable and to seal in moisture. Sebum moves up onto the epidermis through hair follicles. This means that the parts of our body that do not have body hairs also do not have oil; for example, the soles of the feet, the area around the eyes, and the palms of the hands.

The sweat glands are designed to eliminate body waste and toxins and to help regulate our body temperature. They do this by exuding perspiration, a watery, oily liquid, through the pore openings. If we are too hot, then the glands produce extra sweat to help us cool down. The areas that have the greatest number of sweat glands are the palms of the hands, the soles of the feet, the forehead and nose, and the armpits.

The sweat and oil glands work together to keep the skin elastic. The balance between the two determines what skin type an individual has. If the oil glands are overproductive, for example, then the skin will be oily.

The dermis contains within it strong collagen fibers that lie within the connective tissue, as well as fibers of elastin that are more pliable and give the skin suppleness. These fibers also help the skin to expand and, in a young person, it can increase in size by up to 50 percent.

WHY PROBLEM SKIN DEVELOPS

Problem skin develops for a variety of reasons. Heredity may play some part. People whose families suffer from eczema sometimes find that even if they do not themselves exhibit this affliction, they do have excessively dry skin, which may make them appear prematurely aged. If they use soap for cleansing, the problem is exacerbated.

Skin is acidic. This acts as a natural antibiotic, which protects the skin from infection and helps it to retain elasticity. Soap, on the other hand, is alkaline. When the acid mantle is removed by an alkaline substance, the skin's elasticity is compromised. Soap is also drying.

Adolescents tend to suffer from blemishes and even acne. Much of this is attributable to hormonal imbalance but this condition may be made worse through poor diet and stress. Many women well past their teenage years still experience acne at particular times in their monthly cycle and, again, other factors may come into play.

Another possible cause of pimples is that the channels for elimination of waste and toxins have become blocked through the use of antiperspirants or heavy makeup. When this happens, layers of waste build up and finally erupt into a blemish. Pimples may also be an indication that the filtration and elimination of waste products by the liver and the kidneys and the other organs involved in the cleansing processes within the body are not happening efficiently so that impurities accumulate. This can manifest itself in problem skin, since waste always moves outward. Steps then need to be taken to treat the underlying problems.

Some authorities believe that any skin problem is an indication that the individual is not in perfect health, and that for any treatment to work fully one has to make corrections to other aspects of one's lifestyle—such as diet, stress, biochemical abnormalities, medication, allergies, and even skin-care products. The prevailing view is that a poor diet is the main culprit. Too much tea, coffee, alcohol, or foods that are high in preservatives, synthetic flavorings, and chemical residues can give rise to a toxic overload. To compound the problem further, such foods are frequently deficient in vitamins and minerals—all of which are necessary to maintain the health of the skin.

Vitamin C, for example, maintains the integrity of the cell walls and of collagen, the "glue" that holds us all together. Vitamin C also is an antioxidant, which means that it is involved in fighting off certain elements in the body that can cause wrinkling and aging skin. It strengthens the immune system so that we fall prey to fewer illnesses and infections. A diet high in fresh fruits and vegetables will help to keep the body well supplied with vitamin C.

Other vitamins that are vitally involved in healthy skin are B-complex and vitamin A. Someone who suffers from a deficiency of vitamin B_2 (riboflavin) may find themselves with blisters and cracks at the corners of the mouth. If there is not enough vitamin A in the diet, then hair and skin may be excessively dry.

If you address factors of diet and other unhealthful aspects of your lifestyle, then the use of essential oils will be more effective. However, essential oils can help us to start out on the road to well-being by soothing, relaxing, and uplifting us so that we feel better able to make the other changes. What is needed is an integrated approach.

USING ESSENTIAL OILS TO TREAT SKIN PROBLEMS

You can prepare facial scrubs, facial saunas, facial masks, facial toners, and facial oils for your particular skin type by following the directions below and checking the Recommended Oils for Three Common Skin Types box to find the appropriate ingredients.

Recommended Oils for Three Common Skin Types

Dry and Mature Skin (Underactive)
Essential oils: chamomile, rose, frankincense, geranium, myrrh
Base oils:, jojoba, evening primrose, borage
Mask base: honey
Aromatic hydrosol: rose, chamomile

Oily Skin (Overactive)
Essential oils: lemon, bergamot, thyme, patchouli, ylang ylang
Base oil: jojoba
Mask base: fuller's earth or gray clay
Aromatic hydrosol: geranium, orange flower

Normal or Combination Skin
Essential oils: lavender, clary sage, rose geranium
Base oil: jojoba, sweet almond oil, aloe vera
Mask base: gray clay or honey
Aromatic hydrosol: lavender, rose, chamomile

Facial Scrub

An invigorating facial scrub can be made with 1 tablespoon of cornmeal, ground almonds, oats, or wheat bran combined with 1 teaspoon of honey and 3 to 4 drops of an essential oil for your specific skin type. This routine can be done once a week.

Facial Sauna

For a facial sauna, add 3 to 4 drops of essential oil (for your specfic skin type) to a glass bowl containing 1 liter (1 quart) of steaming water. Drape a towel over your head and around the bowl, and hold your face over the bowl for five to ten minutes. Follow the sauna with a facial mask and aromatic hydrosol toner.

Facial Mask

Make a facial mask by combining 1 tablespoon of mask base with 3 to 4 drops of essential oil. Leave on for 10 to 15 minutes and rinse off with warm water. Facial masks are especially effective for oily skin following facial saunas.

Aromatic Hydrosol Toner

Note the difference between aromatic hydrosols and flower waters. Aromatic hydrosols are the true by-product of the steam distillation of plant material for the production of essential oils and actually contain microsoluble components of essential oils. Flower waters often are just water to which essential oil has been added. Thus, the properties of each are quite different.

For a facial toner, use an aromatic hydrosol on a piece of cotton or cloth to remove leftover residue. Put the aromatic hydrosol into a spray bottle and mist your skin to rehydrate or replenish its moisture. Either of these methods will enhance absorption of your facial oil.

Facial Oil

A facial oil blended in a pure botanical base with essential oils will create a nourishing protective barrier between your skin and the harsh environment. Simply add 3 to 5 drops of pure essential oil to 15 milliliters (1 tablespoon) of base oil appropriate for your skin type. After cleansing and toning skin, apply 2 to 4 drops of your facial oil blend.

TREATING SPECIFIC SKIN CONDITIONS

Eczema/Dermatitis

Both disorders have broadly similar symptoms, characterized by inflammation, swelling, and itchy rashes, which often lead to blisters and weeping scabs. The skin is often flaky and patches of skin may be blotchy. The essential oils considered to be the most appropriate for these problems are fennel, chamomile, geranium, sandalwood, hyssop, juniper, and lavender.

Many self-help measures can be tried. Simple application of one or more of the above essential oils in a carrier oil is beneficial. If the eczema is dry, then calendula oil is recommended as a carrier oil, whereas if the eczema is moist, a carrier lotion is preferred. Twelve drops added to 50 milliliters (slightly less than ¼ cup) of the oil or lotion and applied to the affected area every morning or night will relieve the eczema. Which oil is most beneficial depends on the individual, and it is advisable to visit a qualified aromatherapist who can further advise on the best method of skin care.

Products containing lanolin should be avoided, since it is a frequent cause of allergy, as are most dairy products. Infusions made with calendula or chamomile sprayed onto the face can act as a soothing, cooling remedy.

Acne

Acne is a common skin condition that occurs especially during puberty and menopause and is due mainly to hormonal imbalances. Stress and anxiety can also contribute to the problem. When treating acne using aromatherapy, it is essential that diet, exercise, fresh air, and cleanliness are part of the program. Regular and meticulous cleansing, toning, and moisturizing are a prerequisite for the oils to be effective. Oils especially appropriate for acne include calendula, chamomile, juniper, lavender, mint, myrrh, myrtle, neroli, tea tree, and thyme.

An effective treatment for "normal" skin afflicted by acne is a mixture of 50 milliliters (a scant ¼ cup) of soybean oil, 6 drops of wheatgerm oil, and 10 drops of the chosen essential oil. Apply this directly to the skin or use in a compress. For extra-sensitive skin, mix together 25 milliliters (about 1½ tablespoons) of soybean oil, 25 milliliters of almond oil, 6 drops of wheatgerm oil, and 10 drops of the essential oil.

Other treatments include bathing the affected skin with distilled water containing essential oil. A particularly effective mixture is 2 drops each of lavender, juniper, and cajeput in 1 liter (1 quart) of water. Tea tree oil can be applied directly to spots with a cotton ball to stop infection.

Psoriasis

Psoriasis can be treated with aromatic oils although the condition is very difficult to cure. Try mixing together 10 milliliters (2 teaspoons) of wheatgerm oil and 2 to 3 drops of benzoin or cajeput essential oil and applying this to the affected skin morning and night. Lavender and bergamot oils can be used in the bath as well as applied to the skin in a carrier lotion or oil; try 3 drops each of lavender and bergamot to 15 milliliters (1 tablespoon) of base oil. If the skin is very dry and the patches very scaly, a vegetable oil such as sunflower may be better, however, an aromatherapist should be consulted as to the exact amounts and substances to meet the needs of the individual.

Athlete's Foot

Oils that can help in the treatment of this fungal infection include tea tree, geranium, and lavender. The feet can be soaked in hot water to which has been added 2 drops of the essential oil. Alternatively, a small compress with the same oils can be applied and kept in place with a cotton bandage or a sock.

Warts

Onion and garlic oils are effective and can be taken in capsule form. A mixture of raw, chopped onion and garlic applied to an overnight compress is said to remove warts.

Shingles

Start treatment as soon as the symptoms appear. Two drops each of geranium, clary sage, and thyme in 20 milliliters (4 teaspoons) of carrier oil or lotion may be rubbed onto the affected area, and the same number of drops in a small glass of water may be helpful when poured onto the site or applied as a compress.

Healthy Skin Reflects a Healthy Body

It is important to remember that blemished or flaking skin is often the result of some internal disorder. So it is vital to take account of factors such as diet and lifestyle when considering the condition of the skin. Imperfect skin can also be due to hereditary causes. Psoriasis and even hay fever may leave the sufferer with blemished skin.

From a practical point of view, aromatherapy can deal with skin problems through the use of skin care products that contain essential oils for the particular condition. Good care of the skin must involve regular washing with a mild pH-balanced soap or cleanser, and toning and moisturizing with natural and gentle products.

9
Massage Techniques

Since touch is basic to human survival it will come as no surprise that massage is one of the oldest forms of therapy known to humankind. The ancient Egyptians, Greeks, and Romans placed great emphasis on massage, but as a therapeutic system, it is believed to have started in China more than 5,000 years ago, where it was linked with acupuncture and Taoism. Although self-massage can be helpful, it is not nearly so wonderful as a massage from a professional or someone you are close to.

If you go to a professional, you will find that she or he generally specializes in a particular type of massage. You will be shown to a room which should be equipped with a massage table, clean sheets, and somewhere you can change in private. You will be asked to remove some or all of your clothing, since massage works best when there is direct contact with the skin. You may be partially covered with a warm blanket or towel. Some therapists prefer to leave part or all of the body uncovered. Exactly how long the massage will take depends on whether the treatment is local or a whole body massage. The usual length is about 45 minutes to an hour.

Although massage is relaxing, you may find that afterward you feel as if you have had a strenuous bout of exercise, especially where the therapist may have been working to remove years of accumulated muscle tension. This reaction also is affected by how deep the massage was. You are more likely to feel stiff the following day if you had a deep massage than if it was superficial.

This chapter will discuss techniques that will enable you to give someone else a wonderful massage. Who knows, perhaps they'll return the favor!

CREATE THE RIGHT ATMOSPHERE

Wherever a massage is performed, it is important to create the right atmosphere. The place needs to be very warm and comfortable. Make sure there are no drafts. If there are any cold spots, the muscles will find it hard to relax and the "fight-or-flight" hormone adrenaline will be released. Avoid overhead lighting; it can create tension around the eyes and may bring back some unpleasant memories. It is best to work in natural daylight or by candlelight or a soft lamp.

The color of the room can make a difference, too. Pastel shades such as blue, green, lavender, or peach are best for promoting feelings of calm and tranquillity. Matching towels add a special touch, as do flowers or a beautiful painting. Some people find it helpful to play soothing music—but it must be at a very low level, otherwise it will intrude and actually cause tension.

It is particularly important that you eliminate possible distractions or disturbances. The whole atmosphere must be one of peace and quiet. Unplug the telephone and switch off the doorbell. Make sure that the pager or mobile phone is similarly deactivated. Do not let anyone else enter the room.

IMPROVISE A MASSAGE TABLE

Unless you are a professional, of course, you won't be expected to have a massage table, although this is the ideal way to perform a massage. What you do need, however, is a firm well-padded surface. The obvious solution might seem to be the bed, but this has disadvantages. Using a bed means that the person giving the massage will have to bend over too much and that the surface will not be firm enough.

The best alternative is to use the floor. This can be made quite comfortable by supplying a sleeping bag, duvet, foam rubber pad, or thick blankets for the subject to lie on. You can then cover the padding with a sheet or towel. You will want a second sheet or towel to keep the person receiving the massage warm. It is best to kneel when performing a massage in this manner. Make sure that you are kneeling on something soft yourself.

THE APPROPRIATE MASSAGE OIL

In order to mix an appropriate massage oil, refer to the relevant chapters in this book. You also might let the recipient smell the oil in advance to see whether they like it. Although the oil should be chosen with the desired effect in mind, it is more likely that the person will relax with an oil that they enjoy. If the particular smell is unacceptable, then use an alternative oil that will produce the same therapeutic benefit. As a practical point, make sure that the oil is within easy reach so as not to interrupt the flow of the massage.

You will not need a large quantity of oil—enough for one treatment is usually just a few teaspoons. Do not pour the oil directly onto the skin. Instead, pour it into a small dish and then oil your hands lightly, rubbing them together to warm them and the oil before applying your hands to the skin.

MASSAGING THE BACK

It is best to start with the back. If you have had little experience with massage, this will give you the chance to try it out on a large area of the body first. Once you have gotten the feel of giving a massage you will then feel more confident about trying it out on smaller areas of the body. Another reason for starting with the back is that the main nerves of the body radiate out from both sides of the spine and link up with all the internal organs. By relaxing the back you are able to affect the health of the whole body.

How the recipient lies is important. She should be on her front with her head to one side and arms relaxed at her sides or bent loosely upward with the hands placed at shoulder level. If you are using a massage table, you will be standing to give the massage. If you use the floor, then kneel to one side of the person.

Center the recipient before the massage actually takes place, by putting one of your hands on the top of her head and the other at the base of the spine. Keep your hands there for about half a minute. Then move them to the feet, holding one foot in each hand and firmly placing your palms against the soles. In this way, you are sending a message to the person that the situation is safe. It also can be very reassuring to a person who is unaccustomed to being touched.

1. Oil your hands and rub them together. Place your palms at the base of the spine, one on each side. Keep your fingers closed and pointing upward toward the shoulders. Glide your hands up the back in the direction of the heart. Do not put pressure on the spine itself. Keep your hands relaxed so that they can mold into the contours of the body. Move up firmly around the shoulder blades and then draw your hands lightly down each side of the back until you reach the

starting point. (If you find this hard to visualize, think of doing the breaststroke!) Perform these long, slow, and firm strokes several times so that the whole back becomes well-oiled. Make sure it doesn't become too slippery though—about two to four teaspoons of oil will suffice.

2. The next stroke to use is kneading. It is deeper than gliding and helps the muscles to eliminate stored toxins and to separate where they have become bunched together. Move your hands to the sides of the body. There are two methods of kneading. In both methods, use hands alternately.

   For the first method, hold the flesh in the whole of your palm and fingers. Then pull away from the bone, squeezing at the same time. Pretend that you are kneading dough, but don't pinch. Make sure that the whole hand is kept in contact with the person's body. Move up one side of the back and across the tops of the arms and shoulders and then repeat with the other side.

   For the second method, imagine a line drawn down the middle of the area you are working on. If it is the back, then your midline will be the spine. Place the heels of your hands on the midline, keeping your fingers relaxed and outstretched toward the side of the torso. With alternate hands push away from the midline using your whole palm and the heel of the hand. Do not pull up with the fingers. Repeat on the other side of the body.

3. Smaller, more localized movements can be used to go deeper still and to produce a more specific result.

   A *friction* technique is mainly for the back and can be used in a similar way to reflexology in that the back, like the hands and feet, has different zones that relate to particular organs of the body. However, you don't need to know the zones to use friction effectively. Start at the base of the spine. Place each hand on the corresponding side of the body. With the pads of your thumbs, gently apply pressure and move your thumbs in small circular movements for about 10 to 15 seconds. Release slowly and move up along the spine but do not put pressure on the spine itself. As you reach the shoulder blades, work on the muscles in between and above them. Do not massage the shoulder blades themselves.

   Pulling should be done along the sides of the body. Move to one side of the recipient's body. Starting at the hip, work your way slowly up to the armpit and back down again using pulling movements. Point your hands downward to the floor or the table and pull gently upward, using alternate hands. Repeat on the other side.

4. Follow these movements with others that apply some pressure. Put one hand on top of the other. With the whole of the bottom hand make circular movements along the base of the spine and across the hips.
5. Go back to step 1, using long, slow strokes.
6. Use kneading movements on the shoulders.
7. Cup one of your hands, fingers apart, and place the fingertips on a shoulder blade. Press down gently and make circular movements with the whole hand several times in one direction and then several times in the other direction. Move across to the other shoulder blade and repeat.
8. Place both hands side by side and horizontally in the middle of the back. Move the top hand to one shoulder and at the same time move the lower hand to the hip diagonally opposite so that the back is stretched. Do the same in the other direction.
9. Place both forearms across the middle of the back and then gently, but firmly, slide them apart, the top one toward the neck and the lower one toward the base of the spine.
10. Finish the massage by centering the recipient as you did at the beginning. Cover her up to keep her warm and allow her time to "come to."

FACIAL MASSAGE

A facial massage can be wonderfully relaxing, soothing away the worry lines and tension around the eyes and mouth. It can also be used to apply essential oils to the skin in order to treat skin conditions, such as dry skin or blemishes.

Before you apply the oil to your hands, center and connect with the recipient by placing one hand on each side of his head, the thumbs and heels of the hands meeting in the middle of the forehead and the fingers extending downward over the sides of the head.

Apply the facial oil to your hands; use only a dab so that it doesn't run into the eyes.

1. Use your fingers to apply gentle pressure at several points along the jawline, working from the chin to the ears.
2. Use your thumbs to press gently on the hollows on each side of the nose. Use this technique to work your way down both sides along the nose-to-mouth lines, and right down to the center of the chin.

3. With a hand on each side of the face, press under the cheekbones, starting at the sides of the nose and working outward to the ears.

4. Place a palm on each side of the head, with your thumbs lying horizontally along the forehead just above the eyebrows. Work up toward the hairline by pressing gently with the thumbs in parallel lines.

5. Gently sweep the forehead with both thumbs, moving outward from the center of the forehead to the temples.

6. With your index fingers, gently press the tearduct at the inner corner of each eye. Then glide the fingers outward under the eyebrows.

7. Press your hands gently against both ears. Using circular movements, massage the whole of one ear. Repeat with the other ear.

8. To finish, repeat the centering movement you began with.

Materia Medica

10
Index of Popular Oils

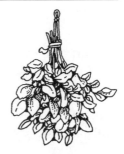

❧ ANGELICA (*ANGELICA ARCHANGELICA/OFFICINALIS*)

Key uses

- Preventing infection
- Digestive problems
- Rheumatic conditions
- Premenstrual tension and menopause
- Coughs and colds
- Bruises, scars, wounds

Family   Umbelliferae (parsley)

General description and habitat   Height up to 2 meters; hollow, ridged stems; large, bright green leaves divided into toothed leaflets; small yellow-green flower groups in large umbels; native of northern Europe and Syria in a variety of habitats; several varieties but the best to use and eat is *officinalis*.

History and folk use   Legend has it that an angel revealed its properties to a monk during a plague. All parts of the plant have been used through many centuries—in China, for colic as far back as the third century. During the plague of 1660, stems were chewed to prevent infection, and seeds and roots were burned to purify the air. Angelica is used in many European countries and China as a medicine.

Essence obtained from   Roots of one-year-old plants

Volatility   Base note

Fragrance   Sweet

Principal constituents   Angelicin, bergaptene, two furocoumarines, phellandrenic compounds, terebangelene and other terpenes (limonene)

Contraindications   Avoid sunlight or ultraviolet light after use because dermatitis may result.

General properties   Carminative, diaphoretic, stimulant, expectorant, tonic

General uses   Rheumatic conditions, indigestion, flatulence, colic, urinary infections, premenstrual tension, menopause, scars, wounds, bruises, coughs, colds, immune system, convalescence, fatigue

✤ BASIL (*OCYMUM BASILICUM*)

Key uses

- Menopause
- Nervous insomnia
- Stress
- Migraine
- Colds
- Hay fever

Family   Labiatae (mint)

General description and habitat   More than 100 varieties; common variety has dark green leaves and is very aromatic; height up to 20 to 50 centimeters; white flowers arranged like a brush on a stem; originated in India, but now grown in many hot countries.

History and folk use   Reached Europe in the sixteenth century. Has been regarded in Europe as symbol of fertility, or even evil or death. The Greeks believed planting should be accompanied by words of abuse! Pliny recommended basil for jaundice, epilepsy, and as a diuretic. Has also been used as an aphrodisiac, and for melancholy and depression.

Essence obtained from   Leaves

Volatility   Top note

Fragrance   Spicy, like aniseed

Principal constituents   Camphor, cineole, estragol (or methyl chavicol), eugenol, linalool, pinene

Contraindications   Do not use in pregnancy. Estragol content may cause adverse reactions in sensitive individuals. Use in low doses or use types that contain little or no estragol (e.g. *O. Americanum Linn* or *O. gratissimum Linn*).

General properties   Carminative, antispasmodic, stomachic, tonic, galacto-genic, uplifting, warming

General uses   Irregular menstruation, menopause, migraine, nervous insomnia, depression, digestive disorders, respiratory problems, stress, anorexia, earache, sinusitis, rhinitis, oversensitivity, neuralgia, poor memory, fainting and migraine, hiccups, poor concentration, indecision, mental fatigue, nasal polyps, nausea and vomiting

✤ BENZOIN (*STYRAX BENZOIN*)

Key uses

- Eczema and psoriasis
- Wounds and sores
- Anxiety, stress, grief
- Catarrh and chest infections
- Arthritis, rheumatism
- Sore throat, laryngitis

Family   Styracaceae (ebony)

General description and habitat The tree is mainly grown in and around Malaysia; height about 20 meters; leaves are oval and hairy; flowers are fleshy, yellow-green.

History and folk use The tree originated in Laos and Vietnam. The ancient Greeks called it *Silphion* and the Romans, *Laserpitium*. Introduced to Europe by Barboza, the Portuguese navigator, it was first known in English as *benjoin* (from sixteenth-century records). Nostradamus wrote about benzoin in 1556. The French used it for inhalations and many medicines have it for a base. In Britain, friar's balsam is a tincture of benzoin compound used for wounds and inhaling.

Essence obtained from Bark of tree

Volatility Base note

Fragrance Heavy, sweet, vanilla-like

Principal constituents Benzoic acid, cinnamic acid, vanillin, coniferyl benzoate, phenylethylene, and phenylpropylic alcohol

Contraindications Not to be taken internally; possibility of allergic reactions, so do skin test first.

General properties Relaxing, sedative, warming

General uses Cystitis, urinary infections, chest complaints, bronchitis, chapped skin, sores and wounds, anorexia, asthma, catarrh, flu, laryngitis, poor circulation, coldness, comfort, coughs and colds, dermatitis, exhaustion, grief, inflamed skin, tonsillitis, throat infections

BERGAMOT (*CITRUS AURANTIUM BERGAMIA*)

Key uses

- Reproductive and urinary problems
- Fever
- Skin eruptions

Family   Rutaceae (citrus)

General description and habitat   Grown primarily in southern Italy, Sicily, and the Ivory Coast (Africa); height up to 4.5 meters; believed to be an orange cross; small, yellowish fruits.

History and folk use   Essential oil has been used since the sixteenth century; discussed in old manuscripts and herbals; believed to have been introduced to the New World by Columbus from the Canary Islands.

Essence obtained from   Peel of fruit (expressed)

Volatility   Top note

Fragrance   Musty lemon

Principal constituents   Linalyl acetate, bergamotine, bergaptene, d-limonene, linalool

Contraindications   Apply with care. Must not be used in high concentrations on the skin. Do not expose yourself to the sun after use because this can cause overpigmentation of the skin and abnormalities.

General properties   Antiseptic, antiviral, antispasmodic, anticancer, anti-inflammatory, analgesic, sedative, cooling, relaxing, uplifting

General uses   Asthma, sore throat, cystitis, anxiety, grief, herpes, ulcers, urinary infections, thrush, psoriasis, oily and open pores, acne, bulimia, colitis, anorexia, boils and carbuncles, eczema, flatulence, gall bladder, indigestion, vaginal itching, loss of appetite

✄ CAJEPUT (*MELALEUCA LEUCANDENDRON*)

Key uses

- Rheumatism
- Stiff joints

- Cystitis
- Bronchial infections, colds
- Hay fever
- Headaches
- Sore throats

Family Myrtaceae (shrubs and trees)

General description and habitat The trunk of the tree has whitish bark, which is fibrous, loose, and can be pulled off in large strips; more than a dozen varieties; grown in Indonesia, Malaysia, and tropical Australia.

History and folk use Thought to have originated from the Moluccas. Used in Malaysia and Indonesia for colds, flu, rheumatism, and cholera. Introduced to Europe in early seventeenth century but was rare and expensive until the Dutch colonized the Moluccas. First mentioned in France in 1876 as having antiseptic properties.

Essence obtained from Leaves and buds

Volatility Top note

Fragrance Very strong, camphor-like, spicy, peppery

Principal constituents Cineole, several aldehydes (e.g. benzoic, butyric, valeric, pinene, terpineol)

Contraindications Not to be taken internally. Use in low concentrations because it may cause irritation. Beware adulterated products, which can cause further irritation (sometimes rosemary, camphor, turpentine essential oils, and colorant are added). An alternative oil to use is naiouli, which does not irritate.

General properties Antiseptic, antispasmodic, analgesic, antiviral, fungicidal, warming, stimulant

General uses   Respiratory problems, asthma, intestinal problems, diarrhea, cystitis, rheumatism, urinary infections, tonsillitis, throat infections, rhinitis, sinusitis, coughs and colds, bronchitis, indigestion, laryngitis

✀ CALENDULA/MARIGOLD (*CALENDULA OFFICINALIS*)

Key uses

- Sensitive skin
- Acne
- Burns
- Varicose veins, broken capillaries
- Painful menstruation
- Arthritis
- Eczema, psoriasis

Family   Compositae (daisy)

General description and habitat   Species of flower native to southern Europe but grows easily farther north in poor soils; height up to 60 centimeters; light green leaves; daisy-like flowers, bright orange to yellow.

History and folk use   "Marigold" is derived from the Anglo-Saxon *merso-meargealla* (marsh marigold). It has been associated with the Virgin Mary and with Queen Mary in the seventeenth century. Was believed that if cut when the sun was at its highest, it would tone and fortify the heart, or that if looked at for a few minutes daily, eyes would be strengthened. Garlands were thought to ward off evil. Marigold poultices were used for the scars of smallpox and other skin disorders. Used today in homeopathy and herbal medicine.

Essence obtained from   Petals

Volatility   Base note

Fragrance   Musky, wooden, rotten

Principal constituents Flavonoids, saponosene, triterpenic alcohol, bitter principle

Contraindications None

General properties Tonic, sudorific, emmenagogic, antispasmodic, anti-inflammatory, fungicidal

General uses Abdominal pain, bruises, varicose veins, gastritis, gastro-enteritis, anxiety, tension, hemorrhoids, cold sores, cuts, wounds, liver tonic, ulcers, indigestion, arthritis, dermatitis, athlete's foot, ear problems, fibrositis, frostbite, impetigo, eczema, menopause, painful menstruation, burns, gout, sprains, acne, chapped and cracked skin, scars, ringworm, stretch marks, rheumatism, chilblains, thread veins

✂ CAMPHOR (*CINNAMOMUM CAMPHORA*)

Key uses

- Circulatory disorders
- Diarrhea, gastroenteritis
- Stress
- Diuretic
- Muscular pains
- Chest infections
- Skin eruptions

Family Lauraceae (laurel)

General description and habitat Related to the cinnamon and cassia trees; height to over 30 meters; native of China, Taiwan, and Japan; evergreen; sometimes grows down to the ground.

History and folk use The Chinese say that it can live for up to 1,000 years; used to be used in mothballs.

Essence obtained from Clippings, wood, and roots

Volatility   Middle note

Fragrance   Mild eucalyptus

Principal constituents   Camphene, azulene, borneol, cadinene, pinene, carvacrol, cineolee, citronellol, cuminic alcohol, terpineol, safrol, dipentene, eugenol, phellandrene

Contraindications   Only to be used for acute conditions because it is highly toxic, especially for those who are asthmatic or allergy prone. Do not use during pregnancy.

General properties   Analgesic, antispasmodic, balancing, sedative, stimulant, warming

General uses   Heart tonic, hypotension, low body temperature, poor circulation, vasoconstrictor, cholera, colic, constipation, diarrhea, flatulence, gallstones, gastroenteritis, digestion, vomiting, worms, anxiety, depression, hysteria, insomnia, irritability, panic, chronic fatigue, shock, stress, diuretic, fluid retention, toothache, aching, antispasmodic, arthritis, fibrositis, gout, rheumatism, rheumatoid arthritis, sprains, asthma, bronchitis, colds, coughs, flu, pneumonia, tuberculosis, acne, bruises, burns, chilblains, fevers, inflamed skin, ulcers, lice, oily skin, wounds

✤ CARAWAY (*CARUM CARVI*)

Key uses

- Digestive
- Painful menstruation

Family   Umbelliferae (parsley)

General description and habitat   Biennial; native to southeast Europe; grows in the wild and in cultivation throughout Europe and temperate Asia; has become naturalized in North America; height up to 60 centimeters;

feathery leaves with umbels of pink or white small flowers; seeds are sickle-shaped and striped and may be confused with cumin.

History and folk use   Archeologists have found fossilized caraway seeds in Neolithic and Mesolithic sites, which shows use up to 8,000 years ago. Used by the ancient Egyptians in religious ritual and in cooking to aid digestion. The Romans chewed them as a breath sweetener after meals and they are often used in Indian cooking. The English common name may have been derived from the Arabic *al-karwiya* or *al-karawiya*.

Essence obtained from   Seeds and crushed fruit

Volatility   Top note

Fragrance   Warm and spicy, musky

Principal constituents   Carvone, carvacol, carvene, limonene

Contraindications   Do not use in pregnancy. May cause irritation, therefore use low concentrations.

General properties   Antispasmodic, carminative, stimulant, emmenagogic, galactagogic, stomachic, warming

General uses   Low body temperature, poor circulation, swollen lymph nodes, abdominal distension, air swallowing, colic, flatulence, gastritis, indigestion, loss of appetite, nausea, stimulates digestion, stomach tonic, worms, irritability, diuretic, fluid retention, dysmenorrhea (painful menstruation), increases flow of breast milk, dizziness, vertigo, aching, arthritis, gout, rheumatism, rheumatoid arthritis, pleurisy, scabies

❧ CARDAMOM (*ELETTARIA CARDAMOMUM*)

Key uses

- Digestion
- Diuretic

- Menopause
- Painful periods

Family   Zingiberaceae (ginger)

General description and habitat   Several varieties; tall herbaceous perennial found in India and Sri Lanka; grows both in the wild and in cultivation in moist soil about 600 to 1,500 meters above sea level; long, spiky leaves; yellowish flowers with purple lips; fruits are ovoid capsules up to 2 centimeters long, divided into three sections containing dark brownish-red seeds.

History and folk use   Has been used in India as a spice and for medication since at least 1,000 B.C. Used by the ancient Egyptians in religious ceremonies and perfumes and by the ancient Greeks and Romans in perfume. It was introduced into Europe by the Arabs through the caravan routes. The name is believed to be derived from the Arab *Hehmama*, which itself was derived from Sanskrit. Hippocrates, Dioscorides, and Ovid all refer to it. Cardamom was added to wine to extract the medicinal properties from the seeds. It was used as a diuretic and to treat epilepsy, spasms, paralysis, rheumatic stiffness, and cardiac disorders. Chinese medicine believes it can treat all intestinal disorders.

Essence obtained from   Seeds

Volatility   Middle note

Fragrance   Warm, spicy, soft

Principal constituents   Cineole, terpineol, limonene, eucalyptol, and zingiberene

Contraindications   Irritation possible, so use in low concentrations.

General properties   Carminative, stomachic, stimulant, antispasmodic tonic, uplifting, warming

General uses Low body temperature, poor circulation, colic, flatulence, heartburn, indigestion, loss of appetite, nausea and vomiting, stimulates digestion, stomach tonic, aphrodisiac, exhaustion, poor concentration, diuretic, painful menstruation, halitosis, headache, sciatica, bronchitis, catarrh, cough

CASSIA (SEE CINNAMON)

CEDARWOOD (*CEDRUS ATLANTICA MANETTI*)

Key uses

- Eczema
- Skin eruptions
- Sexual stimulant
- Scalp complaints
- Genital-urinary inflammations

Family Pinaceae (conifer)

General description and habitat A hardy, long-living evergreen conifer; native of Atlas Mountains of Morocco; the needles form in bunches; yellow male flowers in early summer followed by females; cones have life of up to two years; wood is balsamic, reddish brown in color.

History and folk use Frequently mentioned in the Bible, representing fertility and abundance. King Solomon was said to have built his temple with cedar from Lebanon. Used by the ancient Egyptians for embalming. Subsequently mentioned by Dioscorides and Galen in the first and second centuries as preventing putrefaction. Recognized in the seventeenth century as a urinary and pulmonary antiseptic.

Essence obtained from Wood

Volatility Base note

Fragrance Turpentine-like, sweet, similar to sandalwood

Principal constituents Terpenic hydrocarbons, cedrol, sesquiterpenes

Contraindications Never take internally. Beware adulteration and "cedarwood" from sources other than Morocco. May cause irritation so use in low concentrations. Not to be used by pregnant women or in conjunction with chemotherapy when treating cancer.

General properties Tonic, stimulant, antiseptic, detoxifying, balancing, sedative

General uses Blood purifier, lymphatic congestion, anxiety, shock, hysteria, insomnia, panic, stress, cystitis, diuretic, gonorrhea, inflamed kidneys, leukorrhea (vaginal discharge), premenstrual syndrome, thrush, urinary tract infections, alopecia, dandruff, laryngitis, seborrhea of scalp, sore throat, arthritis, gout, bronchitis, catarrh, colds, coughs, flu, acne, astringent, dermatitis, eczema, insect repellent, irritable skin, oily skin, psoriasis

CHAMOMILE (*CHAMAEMELUM NOBILE; MATRICARIA CHAMOMILLA/RECUTITA*)

Key uses

- Headache, migraine
- Flu, coughs, facial neuralgia, sinusitis
- Hay fever
- Female complaints
- Digestive disorders
- Skin eruptions
- Circulatory problems

Family Compositae (daisy)

General description and habitat Many species, all having finely divided leaves and daisy-like flowers. The sweet variety (*Chamaemelum nobile*) reaches a height of up to 15 to 23 centimeters and flowers between June and August, whereas the wild variety (*Matricaria chamomilla*) can reach up to 1 meter and flowers from May to August.

History and folk use   The ancient Egyptians venerated this plant. Hippocrates dedicated it to the sun because it cured agues (fever marked by recurring chills and fits of shivering). It was established in monastery and domestic herb gardens by the seventeenth century for medicinal and beauty purposes. The Pilgrims took it with them to the New World. In 1656, the herbalist Parkinson advised using it when bathing. Chamomile oil was used up to the Second World War as a disinfectant and antiseptic in hospitals.

Essence obtained from   Flowers

Volatility   Middle note

Fragrance   Apple-like, musty

Principal constituents   Azulene, which is formed during distillation

Contraindications   If there is a real risk of miscarriage, do not use during early pregnancy.

General properties   Soothing, antiseptic, calming, anti-inflammatory, tonic, digestive, sedative

General uses   Fever, digestive problems, colic, flatulence, diarrhea, teething problems, premenstrual tension and other menstrual problems, cystitis, headaches and migraine, earache, rheumatism, skin care, acne, dry skin, eczema, inflamed skin, irritability, loss of appetite, menopause, mood swings, nausea and vomiting, neuralgia, oversensitivity, sprains and stiffness, stomach pains, bruises, aches and pains, colitis, boils and carbuncles, burns, dandruff, depression, dermatitis, enuresis, fluid retention, gall bladder, gum infections, heartburn, high blood pressure, hysteria and panic, immune system, inflammation, insomnia, vaginal itching, kidney infections/stones, liver, lymphatic congestion

✄ CINNAMON/CASSIA (*CINNAMOMUM ZEYLANICUM/CINNAMOMUM CASSIA*)

Key uses

- Flu, colds
- Digestive disorders

- Exhaustion
- Circulatory disorders

Family   Lauraceae (laurel)

General description and habitat   Evergreen trees or shrubs; height of trees up to 18 meters, usually 6 to 9 meters; shiny, ovoid leaves; tiny yellow flowers in clusters; cultivated in tropical countries.

History and folk use   Cassia may have originated in Burma or China. Cinnamon is native to Ceylon. An ancient spice, cinnamon was recorded by the Emperor Shen Nung (2700 B.C.). Most prescriptions in China include the spice. It is mentioned in the Bible and was one of the spices that God told Moses to take with him out of Egypt. The ancient Egyptians used it to ward off epidemics and for embalming. The Greeks and Romans obtained their supplies from the Arabs. The Portuguese (in the sixteenth century) and Dutch (seventeenth century) pursued it, resulting in the colonization of Ceylon (Sri Lanka). The Dutch developed cultivation so that cinnamon became more available in the West.

Essence obtained from   Essential oil of cinnamon is distilled from bark and leaves; of cassia from leaves, bark, and young twigs

Volatility   Base note

Fragrance   Hot, spicy

Principal constituents   Cinnamic aldehyde, caryophyllene, cymene, eugenol, linalool, methylamine ketone, phellandrene, pinene

Contraindications   Possible toxicity, therefore not to be used in pregnancy or with chemotherapy treatment for cancer. Only use when prescribed by a practitioner.

General properties   Tonic, stomachic, antiseptic, warming, detoxifying, antirheumatic, antiviral

General uses   Flu, colds, coughs, pneumonia, sore throats, hemorrhage, low blood pressure, circulatory disorders, acid stomach, diarrhea, indigestion, loss of appetite, worms, depression, fatigue, poor memory, impotence, sterility, fainting, sinusitis, rheumatism, bruises, stings, lice, astringent

✺ CLARY SAGE (SEE SAGE)

✺ CLOVE (*EUGENIA CARYOPHYLLATA*)

Key uses

- Digestive disorders
- Mouth and tooth infections
- Rheumatic pains
- Exhaustion

Family   Myrtaceae (shrubs and trees)

General description and habitat   An evergreen tree that grows best near the sea in tropical climates, usually on islands; height up to 9 meters, generally kept low for harvesting; conical; similar to laurel though leaves are longer and brighter green and have visible dots. Crimson flowers appear at the end of the branches but are picked at the bud stage when they just start to turn pink. Trees under five years old do not produce the spice.

History and folk use   Originated in the Moluccas. Now Madagascar, Zanzibar, and Tanzania are the main producers. The Greeks named the tree *caryophyllum* ("leaf of walnut tree"), which the Arabs turned into *girofle*, which the French use as part of the name they give the spice, *clou de girofle*. The origin of *clou* is the Latin *clavus* from which the English word is derived. The ancient Egyptians, Greeks, and Romans all used cloves. Hildegarde of Bingen recommended cloves for people who feel cold and for those who feel hot (balancing) and wrote that they could be used for headaches, migraines, deafness after a cold, and dropsy. Courtiers in second century China were said to suck cloves to ensure sweet breath before the Emperor.

Essence obtained from   Flower buds

Volatility   Base note

Fragrance   Spicy, vanilla-like, peppery, sweet

Principal constituents   Eugenol, acetyleugenol, benzoic acid, benzyl benzoate, furfural, sesquiterpene, vanillin

Contraindications   Beware of adulterations with vegetable oil. Only use as prescribed by an aromatherapist.

General properties   Stimulant, stomachic, expectorant, sedative, carminative, antispasmodic, digestive, astringent

General uses   Bronchitis, colds, dental abscesses, fever, gum disease, pneumonia, sore throat, poor circulation, acid stomach, diarrhea, flatulence, indigestion, fatigue, impotence, sterility, painful menstruation, earache, vertigo, aching arthritis, fibrositis, neuralgia, asthma, pleurisy, bruises, lice, measles, wounds, sweating, ulcers

⚘ CORIANDER (*CORIANDRUM SATIVUM*)

Key uses

- Rheumatic conditions
- Fevers
- Facial neuralgia
- Toothache
- Nervous facial cramps
- Shingles (face)
- Solar plexus cramps

Family   Umbelliferae (parsley)

General description and habitat   Native of southern Europe, India, North Africa, South America, and former USSR; bright green feathery leaves; umbels of mauve flowers, which later seed.

History and folk use   Thought to be one of the oldest flavorings in the world, its name is derived from the Greek *koris* (bug). It was cultivated by the ancient Egyptians for mixing into bread and the essential oil was used in religious ceremonies. In the Bible it is one of the bitter herbs to be eaten at Passover. In India it was believed to have magical properties and was used in incantations to the gods. Dioscorides and Galen prescribed it. It was used in obstetrics, believed to ease birth and to encourage fertility.

Essence obtained from   Seeds

Volatility   Top note

Fragrance   Spicy, slightly sweet, fresh

Principal constituents   Coriandrol, geraniol, pinene, borneol, cymene, dipentene, phellandrene, terpinene

Contraindications   Possibly an irritant so use low concentrations. Do not take internally except as prescribed by a very experienced practitioner. The wrong dose could be fatal.

General properties   Carminative, warming, diuretic, antispasmodic, analgesic

General uses   Headaches, arthritis, fibrositis, gout, rheumatism, colic, flatulence, indigestion, loss of appetite, poor circulation, anorexia, depression, exhaustion, neuralgia

✆ CYPRESS (*CUPRESSUS SEMPERVIRENS*)

Key uses

- Circulatory problems
- Menopausal symptoms
- Coughs, bronchitis
- Broken veins

Family   Cupressaceae (conifer)

General description and habitat   A columnar evergreen conifer; height up to 45 meters; tiny leaves pressed against branches and twigs; female flowers produce round cones; native to Mediterranean Europe but now cultivated in temperate Europe and North America.

History and folk use   Known to the ancient Egyptians, it was used as medicine and the sarcophagi were made from the wood. Pluto, the Greek god of the underworld, had the tree dedicated to him, which is why cypresses are grown in cemeteries. Its hemostatic properties were known to Hippocrates, Dioscorides, and Galen.

Essence obtained from   Leaves and cones

Volatility   Middle note

Fragrance   Woody, balsamic, amber

Principal constituents   D-pinene, terpineol, cedrol, cymene, tannin

Contraindications   Not to be used during the first four months of pregnancy, or with hypertensives.

General properties   Vasoconstrictor, cooling, anticancer, astringent, antispasmodic

General uses   Varicose veins, broken capillaries, menopause, coughs and bronchitis, frigidity, impotence, asthma, grief, laryngitis, cellulite, change, comfort, whooping cough, diarrhea, glandular fever, gum infection, hemorrhoids, hoarseness, irritability, jealousy, liver, lymphatic congestion, mature skin, menstrual problems, mylagic encephalomyelitis, nervous tension, oversensitivity, oily and open pores, perspiration, poor circulation, urinary infections

❧ EUCALYPTUS (*EUCALYPTUS GLOBULUS/EUCALYPTUS RADIATA*)

Key uses

- Colds and flu
- Bronchitis, catarrh
- Rheumatic conditions
- Genito-urinary disorders

Family   Myrtaceae (shrubs and trees)

General description and habitat   Native of Australia, there are about 600 species; has been introduced successfully to other warm parts of the world, especially Central Asia, North Africa, and California; generally sub-tropical; rapid, tall growth; height up to 27 meters; evergreen, commonly known as gum trees; the leaves of the Tasmanian blue gum are considered to be the best for therapeutic purposes. *Eucalyptus globulus* is used mostly in the pharmaceutical industry because it is rich in eucalyptol and has a very strong odor but because of a rectification process (redistillation of the essential oil) its olfactory richness is lost. *Eucalyptus radiata*'s more subtle odor is generally more pleasant to breathe.

History and folk use   German doctors in the early 1870s were the first to describe its properties. Commercial distillation started in Australia in 1854.

Essence obtained from   Leaves

Volatility   Top note

Fragrance   Fresh, strong, camphor-like

Principal constituents   Cineop or eucalyptol, aldehydes, ketones, sesquiterpene alcohols, terpenes

Contraindications   Must not be used at same time as chemotherapeutic treatment.

General properties   Antiseptic, anticatarrhal, stimulant

General uses   Fever, muscular pain, burns, headaches, colds and flu, coughs, fluid retention, nervous disorders, arthritis, asthma, cuts, urinary infections, tonsillitis, throat infections, stiffness, sprains and strains, sinusitis, rhinitis, rheumatism, neuralgia, mood swings, measles, laryngitis, herpes, exhaustion, cystitis, catarrh, bronchitis, diarrhea, emphysema, fibrositis, inflammation, kidney infection/stones

✺ FENNEL (*FOENICULUM VULGARE*)

Key uses

- Digestion
- Eye inflammations
- Cystitis
- Blood purification
- Bites and stings

Family   Umbelliferae (parsley)

General description and habitat   Native of southern Europe, especially around the Mediterranean, but now found in many other parts of the world, including the United States, Japan, and India. Grows mostly near the sea. Hardy perennial; blue-green feathery leaves; umbels of yellow flowers, followed by seeds.

History and folk use   Used since earliest times by the Chinese, Indians, and Egyptians. Dioscorides and Hippocrates both recommended it for increasing breastmilk. Used by the Romans for its digestive properties, often as an ingredient in a dessert cake. The Greeks believed it helpful for slimming. Hildegarde of Bingen spoke highly of its medicinal properties. First mention of its essential oil was in 1500.

Essence obtained from   Seeds

Volatility   Middle note

Fragrance   Strong, similar to licorice/aniseed

Principal constituents   Anethol, anisic aldehyde, camphene, d-fenchone, dipentene, estragol, fenone, phellandrene, pinene

Contraindications   Low concentrations advised because it can cause irritation. Not to be used by epileptics, children under six years, or during first five months of pregnancy. Not to be used at the same time as chemotherapeutic treatment of cancer. Take care when treating female cancers.

General properties   Digestive, detoxifying, eliminative, tonic

General uses   All digestive and intestinal problems, muscular pain, fluid retention, insufficiency of milk in nursing mothers, stomach pains, constipation, flatulence, bronchitis, shortness of breath, lack of courage, alcoholism, cellulite, flu, food poisoning, hangover, hiccups, kidney infections/stones

✀ FRANKINCENSE (*BOSWELLIA CARTERI*)

Key uses

- Respiratory congestion
- Catarrhal discharge

Family   Burseraceae (resinous trees and shrubs)

General description and habitat   Small tree; height up to 7 meters; grown in the Middle East and Africa; related to the tree that produces myrrh.

History and folk use   Associated with religious ritual, it was one of the gifts from the Magi to Jesus. The Phoenicians had a monopoly on its trade for a long time. Dioscorides and contemporaries recommended the gum for treating skin disorders, hemorrhages, and pneumonia, among others. A sixteenth-century record shows that soldiers were treated with frankincense, and that it was considered good for breast abscesses.

Essence obtained from Gum

Volatility Base note

Fragrance Woody, spicy, lemony, camphor-like

Principal constituents Ketonic alcohol, camphene, dipentene, pinene, phellandrene

Contraindications Not for internal use

General properties Sedative, antiseptic, warming, hemostatic, relaxing

General uses Cystitis, skin disorders, stress, respiratory congestion, bronchitis, aches and pains, wrinkles, ulcers, wounds and sores, coldness, flu, thrush, aging skin, asthma, fast breath, shortness of breath, coughs and colds, catarrh, emphysema, change, fear, grief, hemorrhoids, obsessions, rejuvenation

✻ GERANIUM (*PELARGONIUM ODORANTISSIUM*)

Key uses

- Skin disorders
- Urinary disorders
- Viral infections
- Glandular disorders

Family Geraniaceae

General description and habitat Strictly speaking, these plants should be referred to as *pelargonium*. The true geranium is the herb Robert or cranesbill, which has no therapeutic properties. Pelargoniums originate from South Africa. More than 200 species but only a few are grown for essential oils—*P. graveolens, P. roseum, P. odorantissium, P. capitatum , P. radula*. Main areas include North Africa, Spain, Italy, France, Corsica; other species grown in China, India, and Russia. The best oils come from Réunion and from Egypt. Climate and soil is most important for good quality oil.

History and folk use   No real reference to "geranium" until 1819 when Recluz, the French chemist, distilled the first oil from the leaves.

Essence obtained from   Leaves

Volatility   Middle note

Fragrance   Sweet, floral, rose-like

Principal constituents   Geraniol, borneol, citronellol, linalool, terpineol, esters, ketones, phenols

Contraindications   Beware of falsified oils, which will not produce the right results and may irritate. As stated earlier, look for botanical names and purchase oils from a reputable supplier in consultation with a qualified aromatherapist.

General properties   Vulnerary, tonic, antiseptic, hemostatic, uplifting, warming, stimulant, anti-inflammatory, relaxing

General uses   Urinary disorders, diarrhea, ulcers, viral infections, insect repellent, bleeding, bruises, dry skin, hemorrhoids, inflamed skin, kidney infections/stones, liver, lymphatic congestion, neuralgia, premenstrual tension, other menstrual problems, tonsillitis/throat infections, menopause, anorexia, bulimia, anxiety, depression, mood swings, oversensitivity, eczema, psoriasis, gall bladder, fluid retention

GINGER (*ZINGIBER OFFICINALIS*)

Key uses

- Digestive problems
- Colds, coughs, sore throats
- Rheumatism

Family   Zingiberaceae (ginger)

General description and habitat   Tropical herbaceous perennial; height up to 90 centimeters; enjoys water, humidity, heat; similar in appearance to reeds; yellow flowers with purple lip, orchid-like.

History and folk use   Believed to be native of India; one of the first spices to be introduced into Europe from Asia. Introduced into the West Indies by the Spanish. Jamaica became a major producer, but other producers now include India, Malaysia, Africa, Japan, China, Queensland, and Florida. Used for centuries in the East as medicine and an ingredient in cooking. Similarly used by the Greeks and Romans. Dioscorides used it for stomach complaints. The Romans also treated eye conditions with it. Hildegarde of Bingen, in the twelfth century, recommended ginger for toning and stimulating and also for eye conditions and as an aphrodisiac. It was used in the Middle Ages as protection against the black death. In Dohu, a Pacific island, ginger is regarded as sacred and is added to almost everything.

Essence obtained from   Roots

Volatility   Base note

Fragrance   Camphor-like, lemony, warm, peppery

Principal constituents   Camphene, d-phellandrene, zingiberene, cineole, borneol, linalool, citral

Contraindications   Likely to irritate badly. Always use diluted in pure cold-pressed vegetable oil.

General properties   Stimulant, tonic, antiseptic

General uses   Digestive problems, rheumatism, colds, catarrh, coughs, sore throats, arteriosclerosis, travel sickness, tonsillitis, stomach pains, sprains and strains, poor circulation, nausea and vomiting, lack of confidence, lack of courage, poor memory, diarrhea, flatulence, fever, loss of appetite

Hyssop (*Hysoppus officinalis*)

Key uses

- Coughs, colds, flu
- Asthma
- Bruises
- Sore throats

Family Labiatae (mint)

General description and habitat Hardy, green, and bushy with narrow leaves like lavender and rosemary; height up to 60 centimeters. In France grows wild in poor soil; in Britain often in borders and hedges; royal blue, white, or pink flowers that are very aromatic.

History and folk use Name derived from the Greek *hysoppus*, derived from the Hebrew *ezob* (good-scented herb). Introduced into Britain by the Romans and into America by the early settlers. Has been acknowledged as a medicine for thousands of years. Mentioned in the Bible as one of the bitter herbs to be taken at Passover. Valued by Hippocrates, Galen, and Dioscorides. Used in religious ceremonies, sprayed on worshipers for purification. Used medicinally and in cooking by the Romans, to protect against the plague, and as an aphrodisiac. Mentioned in all the great herbals of the Middle Ages.

Essence obtained from Leaves and flowers

Volatility Middle note

Fragrance Fresh, spicy

Principal constituents Alcohol, geraniol, borneol, thujone, phellandrene, pinocamphone

Contraindications Can have toxic effects and cause epileptic fits if correct dose not given. Never use on sensitive people as it could be fatal. Not to be used during pregnancy. Use only under professional guidance.

General properties   Expectorant, decongestant, stimulant, carminative, sudorific, tonic, antiviral

General uses   Coughs, colds, flu, bronchitis, sore throat, asthma, chronic catarrh, bruises, cuts, wounds, heart tonic, digestive disorders, constipation, gallstones, loss of appetite, worms, diuretic, inflamed uterus, kidney tonic, earache, fibrositis, rheumatism, sprains

❧ JASMINE (*JASMINUM OFFICINALE*)

Key uses

- Infected eyes
- Apathy
- Menopause

Family   Oleaceae (olive)

General description and habitat   One of a genus of about 300; tender and hardy, deciduous and evergreen, shrubs and climbers; flowers generally have a lovely fragrance; most do well in northern climates provided they are sheltered; flowers best after two years from grafting; harvested from July to October—the most fragrant in August and September. Egypt is the largest producer.

History and folk use   One of the principal plants used in perfumes, it was introduced from the East into southern Europe in the early eighteenth century. In the 1830s a jasmine cough syrup was made, although, before that, it was believed to be poisonous. Its therapeutic value has been controversial. In Indonesia one variety is made into a strong tea that is used to bathe infected eyes, and in China another variety has been used for blood purification. Louis XIV had jasmine-scented sheets.

Essence obtained from   Flowers

Volatility   Base note

Fragrance   Sweet, exotic, floral

Principal constituents   Jasmone, benzyl acetate, linalool, linalyl acetate, benzyl alcohol

Contraindications   Not to be taken internally or in the first four months of pregnancy.

General properties   Uplifting, antidepressant, aphrodisiac, soothing

General uses   Apathy, dry sensitive skin, depression, frigidity, impotence, menopause, anorexia, bulimia, childbirth, increases breastmilk, lack of confidence, oversensitivity

❧ JUNIPER (*JUNIPERUS COMMUNIS*)

Key uses

- Rheumatism
- Aching joints
- Fluid retention
- Cystitis
- Eczema

Family   Cupressaceae (conifer)

General description and habitat   An evergreen shrub or tree; prickly; sprawling or prostrate if planted in exposed habitat; height up to 4 meters if a tree; found throughout the northern hemisphere in chalk and limestone; trees are male or female—female trees grow green berries that change to blue-black in the second or third year.

History and folk use   Prehistoric Swiss lake dwellings have yielded up berries. Known to the ancient Egyptians and used by the ancient Greeks to counter epidemics. The Romans flavored their food with the berries and it was used for its antiseptic qualities—recommended for liver complaints and as a diuretic. In the Middle Ages, headaches were treated with juniper, as well as kidney and bladder problems. Hildegarde of Bingen recommended it for pulmonary infections. In Britain it was ascribed with magical properties to ward off witches and to restore youth. In Germany and France juniper was seen as a cure-all.

Essence obtained from   Berries

Volatility   Middle note

Fragrance   Piny, pungent, peppery

Principal constituents   Pinene, borneol, cadinene, camphene, isoborneol, juniperine, terpenic alcohol, terpineol

Contraindications   Avoid during pregnancy. Not to be used with chemo-therapeutic treatment of cancer. If treating severe kidney disorders, use only low concentrations. Beware adulteration with turpentine.

General properties   Antiseptic, depurative, diuretic, tonic, antiviral, uplifting, warming, sedative, balancing

General uses   General poor health, rheumatoid arthritis, insomnia, arteriosclerosis, cystitis, nervous exhaustion, all skin disorders, wounds and sores, ulcers, rheumatism, psoriasis, poor circulation, oily and open pores, obesity, poor memory, lymphatic congestion, colic, fever, food poisoning, cellulite, dermatitis, flatulence, gout, hemorrhoids, hangover, heartburn, indigestion, kidney infections/stones, painful menstruation

🌿 LAUREL (*LAURUS NOBILIS*)

Key uses

- Digestive problems
- Asthma
- Bronchitis
- Rheumatic aches and pains

Family   Lauraceae

General description and habitat   Hardy evergreen; grows well in Mediterranean countries and further north, although is taller in warmer climates;
wild bay trees are common in Greece and south and west France. Has
blackish-green bark; shiny leaves; clusters of insignificant cream-colored
flowers; the female produces berries.

History and folk use   Has enjoyed elevated status—the Greek name for
laurel is *Daphne,* after the nymph whom the gods turned into a tree so that she
could escape from Apollo. The French call the tree *laurier d'Apollon,* dedicated
to Apollo, the god of music and poetry. The ancient Greeks made laurel
crowns for victors in battle, hence poet laureate and baccalaureate. The
Greeks attributed it with mystical powers, as did the Romans. It has also been
believed to be therapeutic for a wide range of ailments—Dioscorides recommended all parts of the plant for a variety of disorders; Galen prescribed it for
liver complaints; Hildegarde of Bingen believed it could cure (among other
things) asthma, fever, migraine, gout, palpitations, and angina pectoris.

Essence obtained from   Leaves

Volatility   Middle note

Fragrance   Similar to cajeput though sharper

Principal constituents   Cineole, pinene, eugenol, geraniol, linalool, phellandrene, sesquiterpene, sesquiterpenic alcohol

Contraindications   Can corrode metal. Don't exceed stated dose.

General properties   Carminative, expectorant, diuretic, sudorific, antiviral,
antiseptic, warming

General uses   Flatulence, slow digestion, asthma, chronic bronchitis, flu,
dyspepsia, rheumatic aches and pains, pediculosis, loss of hair after
an infection

✺ LAVENDER (*LAVANDULA AUGUSTIFOLIA/OFFICINALIS*)

Key uses

- Burns
- Muscular conditions
- Genito-urinary conditions
- Skin problems
- Digestion
- Headaches
- Circulatory
- Emotional

Family   Labiatae (mint)

General description and habitat   Mostly grown commercially in France, Spain, Bulgaria, former USSR, and England; evergreen, fragrant shrub tolerating quite sparse conditions; height up to 1 meter; woody with narrow gray leaves and blue-gray flowers on long stems; several varieties—not to be confused with lavandin, a cross.

History and folk use   The ancient Greeks and Romans used lavender for medicine as well as perfume—adding it to bathwater, hence its name, derived from the Latin *lavare*. In the twelfth century Hildegarde of Bingen wrote a whole chapter on it in her book on medicine; it was grown in monastery gardens in Europe in the thirteenth and fourteenth centuries. Yardley, the perfume company, was making lavender cosmetics and soaps in the eighteenth century.

Essence obtained from   Flowers

Volatility   Middle note

Fragrance   Highly scented, sweet, camphor-like (English lavender), fruity (French)

Principal constituents   Borneol, geraniol, linalool, geranyle, linalyl, pinene, limonene, phenol

Contraindications   If serious risk of miscarriage, not to be used during first four months of pregnancy. Not to be used with chemotherapeutic treatment of cancer.

General properties   Stimulant, tonic, stomachic, carminative, antispasmodic, antiseptic, diuretic, vulnerary, circulatory, anti-inflammatory, balancing, detoxifying, uplifting, relaxing

General uses   Digestive disorders, diarrhea, fever, circulatory problems, cystitis, premenstrual tension and other menstrual problems, childbirth, migraine and headache, colds, flu, aches and pains, arthritis, colic, colitis, earache, motion sickness, allergy, anorexia, boils and carbuncles, bruises, burns, dermatitis, eczema, inflammation, enuresis, fibrositis, anal fistula, sunburn, fluid retention, tonsillitis/throat infection, ulcers, thrush, flatulence, catarrh, coughs, fainting and vertigo, athlete's foot, whooping cough, chilblains, bronchitis, exhaustion, depression, hysteria and panic, insomnia, irritability, acne, aging/mature skin, high blood pressure, hair loss, glandular fever, immune system, urination (difficulty of), shortness of breath, fast breath, liver, cold sores, menopause, stomach pains, stiffness, rheumatism, psoriasis, palpitations, mood swings, oversensitivity, myalgic encephalomyelitis, rejuvenation, oily and open pores, rhinitis, scabies, sprains and strains, palpitations, nausea and vomiting, sinusitis

✌ LEMON (*CITRUS LIMON*)

Key uses

- Poor circulation
- High blood pressure
- Premenstrual tension
- Insomnia
- Colds, bronchitis, sore throat

Family   Rutaceae (citrus)

General description and habitat   Height up to 5 meters; grows mainly in hot climates in the Mediterranean and in California; the least hardy citrus, it can produce up to 1,500 fruit annually; white flowers with delightful perfume. The oils vary according to climate, culture, and soils.

History and folk use   Originating in Southeast Asia, it was known to the Greeks and the Romans, although it was rare. The fruit was introduced into Europe in the Middle Ages. Lemon peel was used as a perfume for clothes and as a pesticide. The Roman agronomist Palladius cultivated lemons in the fourth century and the Arab invaders in the eighth and ninth centuries planted them in the Sahara. The Moorish occupation of Spain led to their introduction in that area. By 1698 lemons were becoming recognized for their therapeutic properties and they were especially sought after for their anti-scurvy effects by the British navy.

Essence obtained from   Rind of fruit

Volatility   Top note

Fragrance   Fresh, sweet, tangy

Principal constituents   Limonene, citral, bergamotine, limettine, diosmine, limotricine, pinene, geraniol

Contraindications   Doesn't keep well, so check date when purchasing. Never use old oil on skin because it may cause a severe allergic response. Do not use with chemotherapeutic treatment for cancer. Avoid sunlight after application and use only low concentrations.

General properties   Digestive, tonic, stimulant, stomachic, carminative, diuretic, antiseptic, bactericidal, antiviral, fungicidal, uplifting

General uses   Poor circulation, anemia, high blood pressure, colds, bronchitis, hyperacidity of stomach, catarrh, coughs, flu, fluid retention, premenstrual tension, acne, aches and pains, gum infections, arthritis, chilblains, cuts, oily and open pores, rheumatism, varicose veins, scabies, neuralgia, mouth and tongue inflammations and ulcers, kidney infections/stones, gout, gall bladder, arteriosclerosis, herpes, warts, thrush, heartburn, liver, obesity, dandruff, diarrhea, glandular fever, mature skin, verrucae (warts), cellulite

✑ LEMONGRASS (*CYMBOPOGON CITRATUS/FLEXUOSUS*)

Key uses

- Slow digestion
- Colitis
- Flatulence
- Skin problems
- Athlete's foot

Family   Gramineae (grasses)

General description and habitat   Grown in the tropics; a grass native to Asia; cultivated in Sri Lanka, India, Indonesia, Africa, Madagascar, the Seychelles, South America, and tropical North America; two types used; *C. citratus* has lemony odor and is less robust (height up to 50 centimeters); *C. flexuosus* is taller with large, loose, gray panicles; propagated by root division; planted in the rainy season; harvested 6 to 8 months later.

History and folk use: Ayurvedic medicine (a Hindu system of healing using mostly herbal medicines) in India has long used lemongrass to combat viral infections, especially cholera. It is also widely used in Southeast Asian cooking.

Essence obtained from   Grass

Volatility   Top note

Fragrance   Fresh, sweet, lemony

Principal constituents   Citral, citronellol, dipentene, geraniol, limonene, linalool, myrcene

Contraindications Consult a professional aromatherapist before use. Sometimes used to adulterate other oils to produce an aroma that smells either of rose or verbena.

General properties Antiviral, antiseptic, stomachic, carminative, digestive, stimulant, uplifting

General uses Indigestion, colitis, oily skin, acne, colic, flatulence, fluid retention, insufficiency of milk in nursing mothers, open pores, scabies, athlete's foot, insect repellent

✌ MANDARIN ORANGE (*CIRTUS RETUCULATA*, SYN. *C. NOBILIS*)

Key uses

- Stress
- Insomnia

Family Rutaceae (citrus)

General description and habitat Member of the orange family but smaller and more spreading with smaller leaves and fruits; delicately flavored; cultivated in Japan and China, the Mediterranean, North Africa, South and North America; essence comes mainly from Brazil, Italy, and the United States.

History and folk use Mandarin oranges have been grown for many centuries in China. No one is quite sure how the name was given to the fruit, though some think that the buttons on the hats of the mandarins at court, which the fruit resembles, inspired its use. The relationship between tangerines and mandarins is also uncertain. Their oils have been used in cooking and in perfumery.

Essence obtained from Peel of fruit

Volatility Top note

Fragrance Sweet, orange/lemon

Principal constituents Methylanthranilate, limonene, geraniol, citral, citronellol

Contraindications Beware adulteration. Do not use on skin before exposure to sunlight.

General properties Tonic, stomachic, slightly hypnotic, sedative, uplifting

General uses Indigestion, flatulence, heartburn, hiccups, anorexia, depression, grief, liver problems, nervous tension, lymphatic congestion, shock, obesity

MARJORAM (*ORIGANUM MAJORANA*)

Key uses

- Insomnia
- Migraines
- Painful menstruation
- Diarrhea
- Mouth disorders

Family Labiatae (mint)

General description and habitat Grows all over Europe and in abundance in Tunisia; known as sweet or knotted marjoram; small shrub with reddish stems and hairy, oval, grayish leaves; height up to 50 centimeters; clusters of pink, white, or mauve flowers.

History and folk use Originating in Asia, it was regarded as sacred in India and Egypt. The Greeks believed it was a symbol of love—young married couples were crowned with its flowers. It was used to enhance the color and texture of hair. Dioscorides prescribed it for nervous disorders, while Pliny recommended it for the stomach and for wind. Hildegarde of Bingen believed it could cause skin problems and was only to be used for healing lepers. During the Renaissance, the herb was widely grown in pots and used for chest infections. Poultices were said to heal jaundice and related diseases. In France, it was prescribed for fatigue and nervous disorders such as epilepsy.

Essence obtained from   Flowering heads

Volatility   Middle note

Fragrance   Similar to camphor, thyme, and cardamom; peppery

Principal constituents   Carvacrol, thymol, borneol, camphor, cineole, cymene, pinene, sabinene, terpineol

Contraindications   Not to be used during first six months of pregnancy, or on young or sensitive people without professional guidance.

General properties   Stomachic, expectorant, sedative, antiseptic, tonic, warming

General uses   Circulatory and digestive problems, nervous tension, rheumatism, migraine, cramps, bruises, thrush, gum infections, aches and pains, colic, stiffness, stomach pains, flatulence, premenstrual tension, anorexia, arthritis, constipation, high blood pressure, grief, hysteria, panic, insomnia, low blood pressure, excessive sexual impulses

✿ MELISSA (*MELISSA OFFICINALIS*)

Key uses

- Headaches
- Depression
- Palpitations
- Insomnia
- Premenstrual tension
- Menopause

Family   Labiatae (mint)

General description and habitat   Hardy perennial native to southern Europe; known as balm or lemon balm; wrinkled, toothed leaves similar to nettle; tiny white flowers; whole plant is fragrant; grows wild and in gardens.

History and folk use   Bees love the plant, hence its name (*Melissa* means "bee" in Greek). The ancients regarded this plant highly. Avicenna described its properties as cheering and other Arab physicians believed it important for easing melancholy and heart problems. It was the main ingredient in Carmelite water, distilled by monks in Paris from 1611. Often used medicinally in France as a digestive and antispasmodic.

Essence obtained from   Leaves and tops

Volatility   Middle note

Fragrance   Soft, warm, lemony, musty

Principal constituents   Citral, citronellol, geraniol, limonene, linalool, pinene

Contraindications   Is expensive and often adulterated with lemongrass or citrus oils. Not to be taken internally. Has been identified as a narcotic. Not to be used in the first five months of pregnancy. Use in low concentrations only.

General properties   Antispasmodic, emmenagogic, stimulant, tonic, uplifting, cooling, anti-inflammatory

General uses   Hypertension, palpitations, colic, dysentery, flatulence, indigestion, vomiting, heart tonic, anger, depression, shock, stress, menopause, problem periods, premenstrual tension, sterility, headache, migraine, vertigo, halitosis

✀ MINT (SEE PEPPERMINT)

✀ MYRRH (*COMMIPHORA MYRRHA*)

Key uses

- Skin problems
- Throat and gum problems
- Sinusitis

Family   Burseraceae (resinous trees and shrubs)

General description and habitat   Native to the Middle East, North Africa, North India; shrubs that are stunted, knotty, and spiky; leaves have three sections and are covered with fluff.

History and folk use   Myrrh was used in religious ceremonies as incense and in fumigations by the ancient Egyptians and was one of the ingredients in *kyphi* (a mixture of scent used in Egyptian rituals). It was also used in embalming. God instructed Moses to take myrrh out of Egypt and it was one of the gifts given to Jesus from the Magi. Jesus was anointed with myrrh after his death. Many ancient texts extol the healing properties of the plant. It has been used for hastening labor and treating skin ulcers and rotten teeth. In the early twentieth century myrrh was still being used in hospitals to treat bed sores.

Essence obtained from   Resin

Volatility   Base note

Fragrance   Camphor-like, acrid, bitter

Principal constituents   Acetic acid, formic, myrrholic, palmitic, triterpenic, alcohols, aldehydes, sugars, phenols, resins, terpenes

Contraindications   Not for internal use or during pregnancy.

General properties   Anti-inflammatory, antiseptic, tonic, fungicidal

General uses   Asthma, catarrh, bronchitis, coughs and colds, hoarseness, loss of voice, thrush, skin problems, eczema, athlete's foot, chapped and cracked skin, dandruff, diarrhea, flatulence, gum infection, indigestion, mouth/tongue inflammation, rejuvenation, ulcers, wounds and sores, wrinkles and aging skin

✄ MYRTLE (*MYRTUS COMMUNIS*)

Key uses

- Hemorrhoids
- Acne
- Bronchial disorders

Family   Myrtaceae (shrubs and trees)

General description and habitat   Evergreen shrub; grows around the Mediterranean; leaves are small, shiny, dark green; fragrant white flowers followed by purple-black berries; height up to 4 meters in its natural habitat.

History and folk use   Venus was believed to have hidden behind a myrtle bush and myrtle was worn in a garland by Jewish brides for luck in biblical times. The ancient Egyptians used to crush the leaves and add them to wine to treat fever and infection. Dioscorides used the same recipe for the stomach, for pulmonary and bladder infections, and for those who were spitting blood. Myrtle was introduced into Britain in 1597. In the nineteenth century its benefits for bronchial infections, genito-urinary problems, and hemorrhoids were recognized. In the south of France women drank an infusion of myrtle to preserve their youth and beauty.

Essence obtained from   Leaves

Volatility   Mid-base note

Fragrance   Camphor-like, peppery

Principal constituents   Camphene, cineole, geraniol, linalool, myrtenol, pinene, tannin

Contraindications   Generally considered mild, but do skin test first to check for irritation.

General properties   Astringent, insect repellent, antiseptic

General uses   Hemorrhoids, cystitis, urinary tract infections, shingles, stings, bites, acne, bronchitis, catarrh, emphysema, diphtheria, insomnia

✄ NEROLI (*CITRUS AURANTIUM VAR. AMARA*)

Key uses

- Depression
- Pregnancy and labor
- Circulatory problems
- Premenstrual tension
- Acne

Family   Rutaceae (citrus)

General description and habitat   The Seville orange tree from which neroli is derived grows in the Mediterranean or in sub-tropical climates; height up to 9 meters; main producers are Italy, France, Tunisia, Egypt, and Sicily.

History and folk use   The oranges were known in the first century but neroli oil was only discovered in the seventeenth century. It is believed to have been named after the Princess of Neroli (near Rome). The Venetians used it liberally to counter the plague and other fevers. In Madrid it was worn as a perfume by prostitutes but this connotation no longer applies and it now is connected with purity. Orange liqueurs use the peel and oil.

Essence obtained from   Flowers

Volatility   Base note

Fragrance   Bittersweet, orangish

Principal constituents   Acetic esters, dipentene, terpineol, farnesol, geraniol, indol, jasmone, camphenes, pinene, nerol, nerolidol, benzoic acid, hydrocarbons

Contraindications   Not to be used with chemotherapeutic treatment of cancer.

General properties   Sedative, antispasmodic, tranquilizing, antitoxic, slightly hypnotic, uplifting, aphrodisiac

General uses   Anxiety, hysteria and panic, anorexia, insomnia, palpitations, bulimia, fatigue, diarrhea, nervous dyspepsia, flatulence, aging skin, broken capillaries, indigestion, childbirth, high blood pressure, colitis, oversensitivity, rejuvenation, nervous tension, frigidity, impotence, depression, fear, grief, shock

❦ NIAOULI (*MALELEUCA VIRIDRIFLORA*)

Key uses

- Colds and flu
- Bronchitis
- Cystitis
- Urinary tract infections

Family   Myrtaceae

General description and habitat   Same variety of the tree as cajeput; native to New Caledonia and Australia; an evergreen with a spongy bark, aromatic leaves, and flowers on a long spike.

History and folk use   The oil is also called Gomenol, as it was first known to be distilled at the port of Gomen in New Caledonia. It was traditionally used by the locals for wound healing, rheumatism, and diarrhea. It appeared in Europe in the seventeenth century. In France, veterinarians use it to treat skin irritations on dogs.

Essence obtained from   Leaves and twigs

Volatility   Top note

Fragrance   Camphor, sweet

Principal constituents   Cineol, terpinol, pinene, benzalhyde, limonene

Contraindications   Although it is generally mild, it can be an irritant

General properties   Antiseptic, antiviral, fungicidal

General uses   Genito-urinary infections, bronchitis, catarrah

✄ ORANGE (*CITRUS AURANTIUM SINENSIS*)

Key uses

- Eczema
- Rejuvenation
- Mouth infections
- Wrinkles

Family   Rutaceae

General description and habitat   The sweet orange tree can grow up to a height of 10 meters; large, dark, glossy green leaves; white flowers; can take up to a year for the fruit to be formed; in tropical areas the fruit is green when ripe, but in sub-tropical and temperate areas it turns orange.

History and folk use   The Arabs introduced the orange to the Mediterranean in about the first century, but it was the Moors who cultivated large parts of southern Spain, including Seville, with oranges. The Romans used orange-flower water to counteract hangovers or indigestion. Oranges were introduced into Britain around 1290 and taken to the New World by Christopher Columbus, who planted seeds in 1493. Oranges are now grown worldwide, including Florida and California. The Arabs were the first to be recorded as recognizing the therapeutic value of oranges.

Essence obtained from   Peel

Volatility   Top note

Fragrance   Orangish, sweet, warm

Principal constituents   Limonene, citral, linalyl acetate, citronelle, geraniol, linalool, terpineol

Contraindications   May cause irritation or browning of the skin after use, so use in low concentrations. Not a long shelf life, so always buy small quantities.

General properties   Antispasmodic, stomachic, digestive, sedative, immune system

General uses   Fatigue, menopause, edema, palpitations, premenstrual tension, stress, colic, constipation, motion sickness, depression, fluid retention, gingivitis, bronchitis, colds, insomnia, mouth ulcers

✂ PATCHOULI (*POGOSTEMON CABLIN*)

Key uses

- Skin problems
- Hemorrhoids
- Abscesses
- Depression
- Fungal infections

Family   Labiatae (mint)

General description and habitat   Herbaceous shrub native to Malaysia but now grown in many places; height up to 90 centimeters; flowers in terminal spikes; harvested three times a year; replanting necessary every three to four years; Sumatra is the major producer, followed by China.

History and folk use   Traditional Chinese, Malay, and Japanese medicine use it as a stimulant, stomachic, and antiseptic. It was the principal remedy for snake bites. Arab doctors used it to treat fevers.

Essence obtained from   Leaves

Volatility   Base note

Fragrance   Earthy, penetrating, heavy

Principal constituents   Patchoulol, sesquiterpenes, benzaldehyde, cinnamic aldehyde, eugenol

Contraindications   Beware adulteration with cubeb (another tropical shrub) and cedar oil.

General properties   Antiseptic, antiviral, fungicidal, anti-inflammatory, relaxing, uplifting, stimulating, rejuvenating

General uses   Anxiety, apathy, depression, anorexia, eczema, impetigo, allergies, fungal infections, cracked skin, abscesses, acne, aging skin, athlete's foot, dermatitis, frigidity, impotence, indecision, wounds and sores

PELARGONIUM (SEE GERANIUM)

✽ PEPPER (*PIPER NIGRUM*)

Key uses

- Sciatica
- Digestion
- Dermatitis
- Colds, sore throat

Family   Piperaceae

General description and habitat   The fruit of a vine found in the moist, low-lying forests in the monsoon area of Asia; also found in the West Indies; in the wild it can grow to more than 6 meters high; when cultivated it is restricted to 3 to 4 meters; thick, dark green leaves; small white flowers, followed by spikes or strings that carry the peppercorns; black, white, and green peppercorns come from the same plant—color depends on maturity.

History and folk use   Long used for cooking and in medicine. Old Chinese and Sanskrit manuscripts mention it. Pliny wrote that pepper was more costly even than gold. In the Middle Ages tribute was paid to kings and princes in peppercorns. Venice and Genoa made their fortunes on pepper trade. The spice was an incentive for the voyages of exploration. It was first distilled in the fifteenth century.

Essence obtained from   Berries

Volatility   Top note

Fragrance   Soft, spicy, hot, piquant

Principal constituents   Phellandrene, pinene, limonene, piperine

Contraindications   Always dilute because it may otherwise irritate the skin.

General properties   Stimulant, stomachic, vulnerary, warming

General uses   Backache, chest infections, sciatica, helps digestion, dermatitis, flu, rheumatic conditions, catarrh, colds, hay fever, headaches, neuralgia

✿ PEPPERMINT (*MENTHA PIPERATA*)

Key uses

- Nausea
- Bruises
- Mouth infections
- Toothache

Family   Labiatae

General description and habitat   Many varieties; native to the Mediterranean and Western Asia, although it grows in all temperate climates; square stems and paired leaves; flowers are purple to white; oil glands in leaves and stems; perennial; United States is the largest producer of the essential oil.

History and folk use   The ancient Egyptians used mint as a ritual perfume and it is referred to in the Bible and in Greek and Roman mythology. Hippocrates refers to the diuretic and stimulating qualities. The Romans used it to help with digestion. The plant was not discovered in England until 1696 and quickly found a place in English medicine.

Essence obtained from   Leaves and flowers

Volatility   Base note

Fragrance   Fresh, strong, penetrating

Principal constituents   Menthol, carvone, cineole, limonene, menthone, pinene, thymol, aldehydes, acetic and valerianic acids

Contraindications   Do not use undiluted or in the bath on its own. Not to be rubbed over the whole body. If used at night, it may keep you awake. Mint remedies are incompatible with homeopathy.

General properties   Antiseptic, antibacterial, stomachic, carminative, antispasmodic, tonic, stimulant

General uses   Nausea, acne, bruises, swollen gums, mouth thrush, mouth ulcers, toothache, abdominal pains, anorexia nervosa, colic, coughing, cramp, painful menstruation, stings, bites, stress

✤ PETITGRAIN (*CITRUS AURANTIUM BIGARADIA*)

Key uses

- Insomnia
- Fatigue
- Acne
- Edema

Family   Rutaceae (citrus)

General description and habitat   See bergamot, neroli, orange.

History and folk use   Also see bergamot, neroli, orange. Plants in the south of France used to be the best source of high-quality oil, which was used for the best cosmetics and perfumes. Today, the main producer is Paraguay, but the product is inferior and used mostly in perfumery and cosmetics. Other oil-producing areas include southern Italy (Calabrian oil is good quality), Egypt, and North Africa.

Essence obtained from   Leaves, twigs, and tiny unripe fruit

Volatility   Top note

Fragrance   Sharp with hint of orange

Principal constituents Geraniol, aeranyl acetate, limonene, linalool, linalyl acetate, sesquiterpene

Contraindications Does not keep well, so buy only fresh oils and do not store for long periods.

General uses Insomnia, fatigue, backache, stress, acne, edema, swollen lymph nodes, deodorant

PINE (*PINUS SYLVESTRIS*)

Key uses

- Flu
- Viral infections
- Genito-urinary infections
- Asthma and bronchitis
- Aches and pains

Family Pinaceae (conifer)

General description and habitat Evergreen conifer tree; known as the Scots pine; native to western and northern Europe and Russia; widespread; believed to be the only north European pine to have come through the Ice Age; height up to 36 meters; short, spiky needles; male and female flowers; cones take two years to mature.

History and folk use Used for the tall, straight masts for sailing ships. In Roman times, pine nuts were used for food and medicine. Hippocrates used pine to treat pulmonary problems and Pliny recommended it for respiratory conditions. In parts of Switzerland, mattresses are filled with pine needles for treating rheumatic ailments.

Essence obtained from Needles

Volatility Middle note

Fragrance   Strong, camphor-like, fresh

Principal constituents   Bornyl acetate, cadinene, dipentene, phellandrene, pinene, sylvestrene

Contraindications   Beware of adulterations. Use in low concentrations because it might be an irritant.

General properties   Sudorific, antiviral, antiseptic, antispasmodic, stimulant, uplifting

General uses   Arthritis, backache, flu, cystitis, bronchitis, catarrh, chest infections, colic, rheumatism including lumbago, rickets, colds, coughing, frostbite, muscle pains, pneumonia, premenstrual tension, stiffness, hay fever, neuralgia, migraine, nosebleeds, sore throat, cystitis, impotence, menopause, painful menstruation

❧ ROSE (*ROSA GALLICA*/*ROSA CENTIFOLIA*/*ROSA DAMASCENA*)

Key uses

- Anorexia
- Premenstrual tension
- Respiratory infections
- Thrush
- Skin complaints
- Nervousness
- Depression

Family   Rosaceae

General description and habitat   Grown in temperate climates worldwide; 250 different species but thousands of hybrids and varieties; about thirty are odorata but only three cultivated on a large scale—*R. gallica, R. centifolia, R. damascena*; the latter is highly perfumed and has the most therapeutic value.

History and folk use   The Greeks and the Romans highly valued the rose, scattering the flowers during banquets, adorning statues, and referring to it in their great legends and myths. The ancient Greeks used roses in religious ceremonies and put them next to mummies in their tombs. Roses were introduced to Europe in the Middle Ages. Monastery gardens cultivated roses for medicinal purposes. It was only in the eighteenth century that the first hybrid appeared. The French have been distilling roses since before the French Revolution for use mainly in rose water. The oil was a by-product.

Essence obtained from   Flowers

Volatility   Base note

Fragrance   Sweet, floral

Principal constituents   Eugenol, farnesol, geraniol or citronellol, linalool, nerol, nonylic aldehyde, rhodinol, stearoptene

Contraindications   Beware of adulteration. About five tons of roses are needed to obtain 1 kg of essential oil and so this product is very expensive. Geranium oil is often used in adulteration, as is geraniol. Adulterated oil does not have therapeutic properties. Be cautious during pregnancy as it has emmenagogic properties. Not to be used with chemotherapeutic treatment of cancer.

General properties   Laxative, anti-inflammatory, aphrodisiac, antidepressant, uplifting, rejuvenating, soothing

General uses   Blood cleansing, nausea, constipation, premenstrual tension, menopause, anorexia, bulimia, nervous disposition, frigidity, respiratory problems, all skin disorders, aging skin, wrinkles, shock, palpitations, headache, migraines, gall bladder, depression, comfort, constipation, coldness, grief, broken capillaries, frigidity, impotence, insomnia, jealousy, liver, sore throats, eye complaints, coughing, shingles, abscess, fever, mouth ulcers, eczema

ROSEMARY (*ROSMARINUS OFFICINALIS*)

Key uses

- Rheumatism
- Depression
- Respiratory problems
- Fatigue
- Headache

Family Labiatae (mint)

General description and habitat Native to the Mediterranean but growing in other warm countries; evergreen flowering shrub; height up to 1.8 meters; dark, linear leaves; pale blue tubular flowers; strongly aromatic; Morocco is one of the leading producers.

History and folk use One of the most well-known herbs, its use can be traced back to the ancient Egyptians. It was sacred to the Greeks and the Romans. Symbolizing love and death, it was associated with weddings and funerals—brides included rosemary in their bouquets. As protection against contagious diseases, it was burned to purify the air and carried around in posies to protect the wearer from the plague. It was sometimes used in place of incense in church. Saxon records mention rosemary for healing and in the sixteenth century it was said to preserve youthfulness. The French regarded it as a cure-all. Hippocrates, Galen, and Dioscorides all prescribed rosemary for liver problems. During the Renaissance it was an essential part of the apothecary's repertoire.

Essence obtained from Whole plant

Volatility Middle note

Fragrance Camphor-like, sweet, fresh

Principal constituents Borneol, camphene, camphors, cineole, lineol, pinene, resins, saponin

Contraindications   Beware adulteration by turpentine, sage, and aspic. Not to be administered during the first five months of pregnancy. Not to be used by hypertensives.

General properties   Antiseptic, stimulant, diuretic, antispasmodic, tonic, uplifting, warming

General uses   Poor memory, poor concentration, mental fatigue, apathy, bronchitis, rheumatism, gout, indigestion, fever, aches and pains, arterio-sclerosis, normalizes high cholesterol levels, anemia, painful menstruation, headaches, migraines, abscesses, dry and aging skin, eczema, acne, asthma, stomach pains, arthritis, boils and carbuncles, catarrh, colitis, constipation, coughs and colds, whooping cough, dandruff, dermatitis, diarrhea, fainting and vertigo, fibrositis, flatulence, flu, fluid retention, gall bladder, hair loss, hangover, indecision, liver, low blood pressure, myalgic encephalomyelitis, stiffness, lymphatic congestion, obesity, palpitations, poor circulation, sca-bies, sprains and strains

❦ SAGE/CLARY SAGE (*SALVIA OFFICINALIS*/*SALVIA SCLAREA*)

Key uses

- Fatigue
- Depression
- Asthma
- Rheumatic fevers
- Sore throats
- Menopause

Family   Labiatae (mint)

General description and habitat   Two of the 448 species of this hardy, ever-green shrub are cultivated for essential oils; native to southern Europe; gray-green, wrinkled, oval-shaped leaves (clary sage leaves are larger); sage flowers are violet blue, clary sage are blue/white; sage is ground hug-ging but can reach 60 centimeters; clary sage is more decorative and can reach 90 centimeters.

History and folk use   *S. officinalis* (common sage) has been grown for centuries for cooking and medicines. The best comes from Dalmatia. *S. sclarea* is mainly grown for cosmetics and medicine. Introduced into Britain by the Romans, its name is derived from the Latin *salver* (to save). The ancient Egyptians and Greeks highly esteemed sage. The Egyptians administered it to infertile women used it and as a protection against the plague. The Greeks believed it could treat loss of memory, deterioration of the senses, and the liver.

Sage and clary sage also were esteemed in the Middle Ages. *Clary* means "clear" (from the Latin *clarus*); it was once used to clear eye infections. Biologists in the 1930s recommended sage for women's problems. Clary sage is regarded as a cure-all (indeed, its Latin name comes from the word "salvation").

Essence obtained from   Leaves

Volatility   Top note

Fragrance   Camphor-like, woody

Principal constituents   Borneol, camphor, cineole, pinene salve, thujone (Clary sage does not contain thujone.)

Contraindications   Sage (*S. Officinalis*) should only be used under the direction of a professional aromatherapist because of its high thujone content. Do not take it internally. Not for use by epileptics, hypertensives, or during the first eight months of pregnancy. Clary sage can be used for self-treatment as it is less toxic.

General properties   Emmenagogic, tonic, stimulant, antisudorific, antispasmodic, blood cleansing, antiseptic, warming

General uses   Abscesses, boils, painful menstruation, catarrh, gum disease, hair loss and other hair problems, palpitations, stress, fatigue, poor concentration, diuretic, kidney tonic, inflamed uterus, sterility, thrush, urinary tract infections, laryngitis, cuts, burns, eczema, asthma, herpes, depression, rheumatism, headaches, menopause, premenstrual tension, gum and mouth ulcers, tonsillitis, animal bites, bruises, sweating, stings

✳ SANDALWOOD (*SANTALUM ALBUM*)

Key uses

- Eczema
- Abscesses
- Cracked skin
- Genito-urinary problems
- Respiratory illnesses

Family   Santalaceae (sandalwood)

General description and habitat   Evergreen, semi-parasitic tree; native to southern Asia; grows best in South India at elevations of 600 to 24,000 meters; height up to 15 meters when mature at 40 to 50 years; depends on nourishment from other trees for first seven years; needs well-drained loam and high rainfall; is an endangered species.

History and folk use   Mentioned in old Sanskrit and Chinese texts, the oil was used in religious ritual; temples and gods were carved from the wood. Imported into Egypt by the ancient Egyptians for medicine, embalming, and ritual. In Ayurvedic medicine (an ancient Indian system of healing) it is prescribed as a tonic, an astringent, to cool down fevers, to reduce inflammations, to treat ulcers and abscesses, to promote perspiration, and to treat mucus discharge.

Essence obtained from   Heartwood

Volatility   Base note

Fragrance   Heavy, sweet, woody, fruity

Principal constituents   Santalol

Contraindications   Beware adulteration with castor, palm, and linseed oils.

General properties   Diuretic, relaxing, antispasmodic, tonic, astringent, anti-inflammatory, aphrodisiac

General uses   Urinary infections, cystitis, fluid retention, anxiety, anorexia, depression, fearfulness, catarrh, coughs and colds, dry and chapped skin, acne, broken capillaries, diarrhea, frigidity, impotence, hoarseness, laryngitis, insomnia, menopause, abscesses, eczema

❧ SPIKENARD (*NARDOSTACHYS JATAMANSI*)

Key uses

- Insomnia
- Stress
- Menstrual problems

Family   Valerianaceae

General description and habitat   Related to valerian; a perennial herb with a straight stem, green leaves with small, pink, bell-shaped flowers; a native of India, Japan, and Nepal.

History and folk use   It is mentioned in the Book of John that Mary Magdalen took a pound of the ointment spikenard, very costly, and anointed the feet of Jesus. In India spikenard was used to darken hair and for promoting growth. Rich women in Rome used it as a beauty aid. Spikenard was also popular with the Egyptians for use in kyphi, a preparation that included other aromatic ingredients such as saffron, juniper, myrrh, cassia, and cinnamon.

Essence obtained from   Leaves

Volatility   Middle note

Fragrance   Warm, musty

Principal constituents   Valerian, jonon, cineol

Contraindications   There are no known contraindications

General properties   Antiseptic, sedative, antifungal

General uses   Stress-related conditions, anxiety, nervous tension, menstrual problems, pregnancy

✤ Tea Tree (*Melaleuca alternifolia*)

Key uses

- Immune system
- Burns
- Infections
- Skin conditions
- Colds and flu
- Mouth and throat conditions

Family   Myrtaceae (shrubs and trees)

General description and habitat   Small tree; height up to 7 meters; small, soft, narrow leaves; cream flowers like bottlebrushes; followed by small, woody capsules set close together; related to the trees that produce cajeput and niaouli oils; grown in a small area of New South Wales, Australia, in dense thickets in marshes.

History and folk use   The early white settlers of Australia used it as a bush remedy but it only began to be studied seriously after the First World War interest peaked around the Second World War but thereafter supplies decreased because of the dangerous environment in which it grew. In the 1970s, interest was rekindled and has increased since then.

Essence obtained from   Leaves and terminal branchlets

Volatility   Top note

Fragrance   Spicy, nutmeg-like, pungent, masculine

Principal constituents   Pinene, cymene, cineole, terpenes, terpinene, alcohols

Contraindications   Use in low concentrations because it is a potential irritant.

General properties   Antiseptic, antiviral, fungicidal, cooling

General uses   Thrush, candida, colds, sore throats, coughs, flu, infection of digestive tract, bronchitis, catarrh, foot problems, verrucae (warts), psoriasis, acne, dandruff, wounds and sores, ulcers, rhinitis, perspiration, oily and open pores, myalgic encephalomyelitis, mouth infections/ulcers, sinusitis, herpes, gum infections, boils and carbuncles, chapped and cracked skin, cold sores, cuts, cystitis, glandular fever, immune system, vaginal itching

✭ THUJA (*THUJA* SPP)

Key uses

- Psoriasis
- Alopecia
- Acne

Family   Cupressaceae (conifer)

General description and habitat   A type of evergreen tree/shrub; native to North America, Japan, China, and Korea; known as white cedar; small, slow growing; leaves pressed closely to stem; male and female flowers on same tree; small, scaly cones; strongly aromatic.

History and folk use   *Thuja* is the Latinized form of the Greek *thuo* (to sacrifice). It was grown in Cyrene near the Temple of Jupiter/Ammon and was burned to honor the gods. Its bark was used to sculpt religious images. Leaves and bark were made into a poultice by the American Indians and used for rheumatic conditions and infused to make a decoction for drinking to combat viral infections. Hahnemann (1755–1843), who founded homeopathy, introduced its therapeutic qualities into Europe. In the nineteenth century, its healing powers were extolled.

Essence obtained from   Leafy young twigs

Volatility   Top note

Fragrance   Fresh, pungent

Principal constituents   Pinene, borneol, bornyl acetate, thujone, fenchone, fenone

Contraindications   Not for self treatment because of possible toxicity. Consult an aromatherapist. Not to be taken internally.

General properties   Antirheumatic, antiseptic

General uses   Psoriasis of scalp, weeping skin, hair loss, acne, severe infection, tumors, warts, urinary problems

THYME (*THYMUS* SPP)

Key uses

- Asthma
- Flu, colds
- Fever
- Skin problems
- Backache
- Rheumatism

Family   Labiatae (mint)

General description and habitat   Native to Europe, especially the Mediterranean; now spread worldwide, to America and even Iceland; some provide groundcover, others can grow up to 30 centimeters; leaves of all species are aromatic, more so in cultivated species; those grown in warm climates are more powerfully scented than those in colder climates; depending on the variety, flowers range from white to pale pink, lilac, and deep red.

History and folk use   Believed to have been used as long ago as 3500 B.C. by the Sumerians. Known to the ancient Egyptians as *tham*, it was used in embalming. The Greeks used "white" thyme for digestive purposes and for offering to the gods. The Romans used the plant medicinally, e.g. for epilepsy, relaxation, headaches, and snake bites. Burning it outside houses was said to keep dangerous reptiles away. The Romans also believed thyme cured melancholy and imbued bravery—soldiers would bathe in it before confronting the enemy. During the Crusades, ladies embroidered it on their knights' scarves. Hildegarde of Bingen recommended it for plague, paralysis, leprosy, and body lice. In the seventeenth century, it was believed to be a brain strengthener and in the eighteenth century, it was included in many medical preparations. During the First World War, it was used as a disinfectant in hospitals.

Essence obtained from   Flowers, leaves

Volatility   Middle note

Fragrance   Light, fresh, slightly musty

Principal constituents   Thymol, carvacrol, borneol, cineole, linalool, menthone, cymene, pinene, triterpenic acid

Contraindications   Not to be used by children, hypertensives, or pregnant women. Use only with professional guidance.

General properties   Tonic, stimulant, stomachic, digestive, antispasmodic, antiviral, warming

General uses   Poor circulation, anemia, gout, low blood pressure, anorexia, urinary tract infections, mouth infections, rheumatism, nervous exhaustion, colds, coughs, poor memory, arthritis, asthma, whooping cough, glandular fever, rhinitis, aches and pains, boils, carbuncles, dandruff, depression, flatulence, immune system, irritability, myalgic encephalomyelitis, scabies, sinusitis, wounds and sores, flu, pneumonia, halitosis, stings and bites, bruises, indigestion, anemia, poor menstruation, liver tonic, mumps, hair loss

✿ VERBENA (*LIPPIA CITRIODORA* SYN. *ALOYSIA CITRIODORA*)

Key uses

- Acne
- Stomach problems
- Depression

Family   Verbenaceae

General description and habitat   Perennial, deciduous shrub; slender with height up to 1.5 meters; native of South America; long, pointed, pale green leaves; tubular purple flowers that grow in clusters; whole plant smells of lemon.

History and folk use   Verbena was introduced into North Africa, India, Australia, the Caribbean islands, and Réunion, reaching Europe in about 1760. Its original botanical name was after Augustin Lippi, a seventeenth-century Italian naturalist. The plant is now renamed *Aloysia citriodora*. It was first described in about 1784 as a fortifier and normalizer of the nervous system.

Essence obtained from   Leaves and stalks

Volatility   Top note

Fragrance   Fresh, lemony, hot, bitter, subtle

Principal constituents   Citral, caryophyllene, cineole, geraniol, limonene, linalool, methylheptenone, nerol, terpineol

Contraindications   The true oil is expensive and is therefore often adulterated. Can cause skin irritations in some people.

General uses Appetite (lack of), depression, acne, dermatitis, nervous system, flatulence, dizziness, hysteria

WINTERGREEN (*GAULTHERIA PROCUMBENS*)

Key uses

- Rheumatic conditions
- Muscular pains
- Gout

Family Ericaceae

General description and habitat One of 200 species; evergreen flowering shrub; native to northern United States and Canada; height about 30 centimeters; grows in mountainous regions or on sandy, deserted plains; large, oval, glossy, toothed leaves; flowers are white or pink bells that droop; berries are aromatic and bright red.

History and folk use Also known as partridge berry and checkerberry, it has been used for hundreds of years by the American Indians for such ailments as pain or fever, or to feed to their animals. In the nineteenth century it was considered a cure-all.

Essence obtained from Leaves

Volatility Middle note

Fragrance Aromatic, camphor-like, vanilla-like

Principal constituents Methylsalicylate, ketone, alcohol

Contraindications Beware commercial preparations, which often have a synthetic base or are adulterated with other oils, causing disappointing results.

General properties Diuretic, stimulant, emmenagogic, antirheumatic

General uses Rheumatic conditions, gout, stiffness, rejuvenating, muscular pains, boils, edema, cellulite

YLANG-YLANG (*CANANGA ODORATA*)

Key uses

- Circulatory problems
- Stress
- Aphrodisiac

Family Annonaceae (tropical trees and shrubs)

General description and habitat Originating in the Philippines, these trees have now spread throughout tropical Asia; small, but can reach up to 30 meters; branches droop like a willow; large, oval, shiny leaves; flowers in clusters, starting out green but turning yellow about 20 days later, highly perfumed; profusion of flowers in the rainy season; greenish fruit; in recent years production has been declining and inferior quality oils from other varieties are being marketed.

History and folk use Filipinos used the flowers to make a pomade, which they rubbed on their bodies to ward off fever in the rainy season. The islanders also mixed the flowers with coconut oil to protect their hair from the saltwater when swimming. It kept their skin healthy and helped to counter insect and snake bites. Cananga (ylang-ylang) oil was used in nineteenth-century Europe as a hair oil. It was discovered to have therapeutic properties in the late nineteenth to early twentieth century.

Essence obtained from Flowers

Volatility Base note

Fragrance Sweet, narcissus-like, hyacinth-like

Principal constituents Pinene, benzoic acid, cadinene, caryophyllene, cresol, eugenol, isoeugenol, linalyl acetate, linalyl benzoate, linalool, geraniol

Contraindications   Beware falsification with other oils. High concentrations may cause headaches or nausea.

General properties   Stimulant, relaxing, antiseptic, aphrodisiac

General uses   Poor circulation, anemia, gout, low blood pressure, anorexia, urinary infections, mouth infections, rheumatism, nervous exhaustion, colds, coughs, poor memory, arthritis, asthma, whooping cough, glandular fever, rhinitis, boils and carbuncles, dandruff, depression, flatulence, fluid retention, immune system, irritability, loss of appetite, mouth infections/ulcers, myalgic encephalomyelitis, scabies, sinusitis, wounds and sores

Index of Ailments

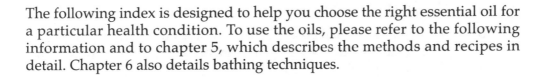

The following index is designed to help you choose the right essential oil for a particular health condition. To use the oils, please refer to the following information and to chapter 5, which describes the methods and recipes in detail. Chapter 6 also details bathing techniques.

❧ How to Use Essential Oils

Bath (2 to 10 drops)

- Run bathwater as usual, add the drops of essential oil, and swirl the water to disperse.
- If you have sensitive skin, dilute in a small amount (5 millimeters) of a base oil such as jojoba and add to the water.
- Keep the bathroom door closed to retain the aroma in the bathroom.
- Avoid using soaps or body shampoos when using essential oils.

Hand or foot bath (3 to 5 drops)

- Add essential oil to a bowl of warm water and swirl.
- Soak hands or feet for ten to fifteen minutes.

Sitz bath (2 to 3 drops)

- Add essential oils to the bath and swirl the water to disperse.
- Blend in a base oil if you have sensitive skin.
- Keep the bathroom door closed to retain the aroma.
- Avoid using soaps when using essential oils.

Gargle (1 to 2 drops)

- Add essential oil to a teaspoon of honey.
- Dissolve this blend in 30 milliliters (2 tablespoons) of warm water.
- Gargle a small amount and spit out.
- *Do not swallow.*

Inhalation (1 to 2 drops)

- Do not inhale directly from bottle.
- Put 1 or 2 drops on a handkerchief or a paper towel.
- Inhale by taking deep breaths.

Steam inhalation (1 to 2 drops)

- Add 1 or 2 drops to a small bowl of steaming water.
- Cover your head and the bowl with a towel, making sure you are at a comfortable distance above the bowl.
- Inhale deeply with your nose, keeping your eyes closed.
- Raise the towel and take a deep breath through your mouth, then lower the towel and inhale.
- Continue this procedure until the smell is gone.

Massage oil (refer to chapter 5)

Compress (3 to 5 drops)

- Add the drops of essential oil to a small bowl of water.
- Soak a piece of cotton or any other absorbent material large enough to cover the area to be treated.
- Use 100 percent unbleached natural material for maximum effect.
- Squeeze out the compress gently so that it is not dripping.
- Place over the affected area, using plastic wrap or a bandage to secure it in place.
- Leave in place for 1 to 2 hours.

Room fragrance

- Buy a diffuser (many types are available). Most rely on gentle heat to activate the essential oils. Make sure you have water in the bowl of the diffuser to keep the essential oil from burning.

- Add essential oil to potpourri or dried flowers.
- Special rings to use with table lamps are now available.

✖ ABSCESS

This is an accumulation of pus in a particular part of the body caused by an infection. It is painful to touch because of the increase of white blood cells in the area, which are there to fight off the infection by liquefying the invading germs. The abscess eventually comes to a head and ruptures. It may be accompanied by a raised temperature. Abscesses are often a sign of being run down (exhaustion) or of a poor diet. They also often occur at times of hormonal change or in people who suffer from some other complaint such as diabetes or acne.

Recurrent, multiple, or large abscesses should receive immediate medical attention because antibiotics might be needed. Medical attention should also be sought if the abscess forms in a joint or gland or in the chest or abdominal cavity. Don't wait until it bursts.

Oils to use

Bergamot, chamomile, frankincense, tea tree

How to use

Baths, massage, compress

✖ ACNE

This common skin condition is caused by excessive production of sebum. When sebaceous glands become blocked and infected, pimples appear, usually on the face, back, and chest.

Acne usually occurs in adolescence due to hormonal changes but may also, in women, be caused by the hormones involved in menstruation or menopause. Other factors may be poor diet, constipation (poor elimination), stress, and anxiety. It is important to have sufficient exercise and fresh air and efforts should be made to improve the diet. Cleanliness is vital. Try to use products that do not dry out the skin such as gentle soaps and aftershave.

Oils to use

Bergamot, cajeput, chamomile, frankincense, lavender, lemongrass, juniper, sandalwood, tea tree, myrrh

How to use

Facial oils, skin tonics, massage, baths

Addictions

There are many forms of addiction. When treating an addiction, it is vital to look at the underlying causes because unless these are dealt with, any form of treatment will have little lasting value. For severe addictions you should seek medical help. If the basis for the addiction is emotional, counseling and psychotherapy should help. Essential oils can alleviate the symptoms of withdrawal and help to make it bearable.

Oils to use

Depression—Bergamot, chamomile, geranium, lavender, patchouli, rose, sandalwood, ylang-ylang
For uplifting—Clary-sage, jasmine
Nervous tension—Basil, marjoram, neroli, rose, mandarin orange
Irritability—Chamomile, cypress, lavender, thyme
Insomnia—Chamomile, marjoram, rose, ylang-ylang
Lack of confidence—Ginger, jasmine
Indecision—Basil, patchouli
Loneliness—Benzoin
Immune system—Chamomile, lemon, thyme

How to use

Baths, massage, room fragrance

Allergies

An allergy is caused by the immune system overreacting to internal or external substances that may not actually be harmful. Sometimes this is caused by the inability of the liver to detoxify the body, perhaps because of toxic overload, so that the immune system becomes hypersensitive. Food allergies also may be caused by too early an introduction of such foods as dairy products, wheat, eggs, and sugar to an infant. Breastfeeding has been proven to reduce the risk of allergies later in life.

Symptoms of allergies include asthma, catarrh, eczema, urticaria, constipation, stomach pains, headaches, tiredness, and hyperactivity. It may be necessary to embark on an elimination diet, but you must seek medical supervision and nutritional expertise first.

Oils to use

Chamomile, lavender, patchouli, lemon

How to use

Baths, massage, compress

ALOPECIA (SEE HAIR LOSS)

ANEMIA

This blood disorder is due to insufficient hemoglobin in the blood. Hemoglobin carries oxygen and a lack of hemoglobin results in a corresponding lack of oxygen. The symptoms of this are dizziness, tiredness, breathlessness, palpitations, brittle nails, and poor appetite.

The underlying causes should be identified. Anemia may be due to an iron deficiency or to a deficiency in the B vitamins, especially folic acid and B_{12}. The deficiency might be brought on by excessive menstrual bleeding, pregnancy, or blood loss after surgery.

You can address the deficiency through diet by eating plenty of foods rich in iron and in the B vitamins. Increase your intake of vitamin C because this enhances the absorption of iron. Reduce your consumption of coffee. Essential oils will help to revitalize you.

Oils to use

Chamomile, lemon, peppermint, rosemary, lavender, melissa

How to use

Baths, massage, inhalation

❧ Anorexia and Bulimia

Usually disorders that affect adolescent girls, anorexia and bulimia seem to be on the increase in boys. Anorectics feel a complete aversion to food, which results in severe weight loss that can ultimately cause death due to starvation. The bulimic will often gorge and then induce vomiting. These are complex conditions with many possible causes—family disharmony or pressures, feelings of inadequacy, social pressures to look slim. They can even be caused by a zinc deficiency due to eating junk food.

Expert help is vital. Counseling is essential. Nutritional supplements can help ensure adequate vitamin and mineral intake. Small, attractive, flavorful meals may entice the reluctant eater. Essential oils can help, particularly when coupled with massage so that the person can be helped to accept her or his body. They may also stimulate appetite.

Oils to use

Marjoram, thyme, melissa

How to use

Massage; neat on back of hands, soles and tops of feet, and solar plexus

❧ Anxiety

We all feel anxious at some time or another in our lives. Certain conditions, particularly sudden changes, can trigger anxiety. These stressful events take their toll if they come too quickly at us, or if we do not find adequate ways of dealing with them. Anxiety can manifest itself in a number of ways, including insomnia, irritability, headaches, and digestive disorders. More seriously, hypertension can result. This is because adrenaline, the fight-or-flight hormone, is continually being produced in response to our anxiety.

It may be necessary to seek expert help in the form of counseling or therapy if you are overwhelmed by the feeling and are unable to resolve it. For free-floating anxiety to be overcome, the roots of the disorder need to be uncovered before any improvement can take place. Therapeutic oils can help to relax you and lighten any accompanying depression.

Oils to use

Chamomile, clary-sage, geranium, jasmine, lavender, marjoram, patchouli, rose

How to use

Massage, baths

✄ ARTHRITIS

This term covers a number of disorders, all of which involve inflammation of the joints. The types that are usually meant are osteoarthritis and rheumatoid arthritis. Osteoarthritis is generally considered to be a painful result of general wear and tear in the aging process. Rheumatoid arthritis is a disease of the connective tissue that results in swelling, pain in the joints, fatigue, and fever.

Diet can help to some extent. Avoid meat, coffee, alcohol, tobacco, and fats. Eat foods that are high in calcium, magnesium, and vitamin C. Exercise is particularly beneficial for osteoarthritis. Essential oils can help to relieve the pain. Some oils that are beneficial for osteoarthritis should not be used for rheumatoid arthritis because rheumatoid arthritis is an auto-immune disease and some of the oils stimulate the immune system.

Oils to use for osteoarthritis

Lavender, chamomile, cypress, pine, juniper, eucalyptus, coriander, lemon, rosemary, marjoram, ginger

Oils to use for rheumatoid arthritis

Lavender, cypress, pine, juniper, coriander, marjoram, ginger

How to use

Compresses, baths, massage, rub affected area with massage oil

✖ ASTHMA

The airways of the upper respiratory tract are affected by this disorder. The bronchi of the lungs go into spasm and the airways constrict, resulting in a shortage of breath, wheezing, choking, and coughing. Asthma usually starts in childhood and is generally thought to afflict those people who are emotionally sensitive, although there are a number of causes, such as food allergies, dust mites, feathers, animals, cigarette smoke, molds, grasses, and pollen.

You should always seek medical advice for this condition. Exercise, especially swimming, is beneficial. Care must be taken when using essential oils. Some aromatherapists maintain that no oils should be applied and that herbal tisanes are more appropriate than essential oils. Steam inhalations should not be given because they can trigger an attack.

Oils to use

Benzoin, cajeput, cypress, eucalyptus, frankincense, lavender, lemon, myrrh, peppermint, rosemary, thyme

How to use

Baths, massage, chest rubs

✖ ATHLETE'S FOOT

This condition is caused by a fungal infection. The flesh between the toes becomes moist, flaky, and itchy. Affected toenails become brittle. Usually it is caught in gymnasiums or locker rooms and from bathroom floors. It is important to keep your feet fresh by bathing them daily. Wear only cotton socks and leather or canvas shoes and wear different shoes each day. Avoid sugar in your diet as well as alcohol. Consume garlic and onion and foods rich in beta-carotene such as green leafy vegetables. Foot baths with essential oils are particularly helpful.

Oils to use

Tea tree, geranium, lavender, myrrh, calendula

How to use

Foot baths, neat oil dabbed on with cotton ball, compress

✣ Backache (See Lumbago)

✣ Blisters

Fluid accumulates under an area of skin, perhaps because of rubbing from shoes, or from injuries such as burns, scalds, or insect stings. Sometimes blisters are a result of eczema, impetigo, herpes, or chicken pox. The blister usually bursts and in order to avoid infection of the underlying skin, the area should be kept clean.

Oils to use

Benzoin, lavender

How to use

Dab on with cotton wool

✣ Boils

You may suffer from these if you are run down or have been consuming a particularly rich diet. Boils are the result of the body attempting to eliminate toxins. If the exit from the body is blocked up or if the blood and lymph are circulating poorly, the toxins can build up in a hair follicle. If you are suffering from frequent boils, then you should seek medical advice because this may indicate an underlying condition such as diabetes. Get plenty of exercise and include parsley, raw spinach, and plenty of vitamin C in your diet. Avoid dairy products, except live yogurt.

Oils to use

Chamomile, lavender, lemon, rose, tea tree

How to use

Baths, compresses, dab on with cotton wool

✤ Bronchitis

There are two sorts of bronchitis—acute and chronic. Acute bronchitis is usually due to the persistence of a bacterial or viral infection such as a cold. It can be particularly serious in babies and the elderly. Chronic bronchitis is usually due to long-term irritation of the bronchial lining—perhaps by cigarette smoke or damp or dusty environments. It is important that the mucus is coughed up so as to clear any infection that exists. Bronchitis is usually accompanied by chest pain and fever. Drinking herbal teas, eating to build up the immune system, avoiding of dairy products, and giving up smoking are all important in the treatment.

Oils to use

Cedarwood, eucalyptus, frankincense, lavender, lemon, myrrh, rosemary, sandalwood, tea tree, thyme, pine, wintergreen

How to use

Chest rubs, poultices, baths, humidifier, steam inhalation, massage

✤ Bruises

A bruise is simply bleeding under the skin as a result of an injury. Sometimes there is pain, especially if the bruise is located above a bone since the blood-congested tissues stretch more tightly over the bone. Some people are more prone to bruising than others—particularly the elderly, anemic, and obese. If left alone, most bruises will heal themselves.

Oils to use

Chamomile, calendula, lavender, cypress, geranium, marjoram

✤ Bulimia (See Anorexia and Bulimia)

❧ BURNS

Essential oils are particularly useful for burns. Gattefosse, you will recall, plunged his hand into lavender oil after burning his hand and was astonished to find how quickly the injury healed.

Burns are caused by heat—either dry (as in the case of fire, the sun, or electricity) or moist (such as steam and boiling liquids). Damage is caused to the skin and there is considerable pain at the nerve endings. Serious burns must always receive medical attention.

Essential oils have antibacterial and antiviral properties that help to keep infection at bay. They also help to stimulate new skin growth.

Oils to use

Lavender, eucalyptus, calendula, clary sage

How to use

Neat (lavender oil), baths, compresses

❧ CANDIDA

This yeast-like fungus grows in the intestines, mouth, and vagina in warm, moist, sugary conditions. Pregnant women and diabetics are prone to this condition, as are those whose immune systems are suppressed, such as those with AIDS. Too much reliance on antibiotics can also cause candida because antibiotics destroy not only harmful bacteria but also the helpful bacteria that keep conditions stable in the body and prevent this fungus from flourishing.

It is easy to overlook candidiasis as a disease because its symptoms can be attributed to other causes. The main symptoms are headaches, fatigue, allergies, constipation, cystitis, depression, bloating, and diarrhea. Oral thrush is easier to diagnose because the tongue and inside of the mouth is usually covered in white spots and there may be soreness and a burning feeling.

If you are suffering from candida, avoid sugar in any form, as well as alcohol and yeast-containing foods such as bread, mushrooms, cheese, and yeast spreads. Eat plenty of fresh vegetables, especially garlic and onions. Increase your intake of live, natural yogurt.

Oils to use

Tea tree and eucalyptus

How to use

Baths, compresses, massage, gargle

❧ CATARRH

Catarrh is the excessive production of mucus in the lungs, larynx, nose, and sinuses. It often occurs as a result of a cold or hay fever or because of general overload in the body. The condition can be painful because the mucous membranes become inflamed. Smoking should be stopped. Tea, coffee, chocolate, dairy products, and other foods that stimulate mucus production should be avoided. Boost your intake of raw foods.

Oils to use

Benzoin, chamomile, eucalyptus, frankincense, hyssop, mint, niaouli, pine, clary sage

How to use

Baths, steam inhalation, room fragrance

❧ CELLULITIS

To the women who suffer from this problem, cellulitis is much more than a beauty defect. In Europe cellulitis is actually recognized as a medical condition. High levels of estrogen encourage the body tissues to retain water, which then becomes interspersed with fat cells so that the skin assumes an "orange peel" texture. Cellulite is usually found on the thighs, buttocks, and hips. Sometimes it even appears on the stomach, upper arms, and the back of the neck.

Probable causes include malfunctioning of the endocrine glands, which means excessive amounts of estrogen are being produced; poor digestion of food; constipation; nervous disorders; bad posture; contraceptive pills; and smoking.

Adjusting your diet is important. Consume plenty of raw, fresh foods, especially those high in vitamin C. Get plenty of exercise. Learn a relaxation technique.

Oils to use

Cypress, lavender, lemon, juniper, rosemary

How to use

Baths, massage, rub and knead affected areas with massage oil

Chilblains

The toes, fingers, and backs of the legs are particularly prone to this disorder because these parts of the body are the most exposed to cold. The condition is also exacerbated by poor circulation. Symptoms are patches of inflamed reddish-blue discolored skin, which itch and can become ulcerated. In cold weather you should always ensure that you and your children are adequately protected against the cold, being especially careful to dry your hands and feet properly.

Oils to use

Cypress, lavender, tea tree, lemon, sandalwood

How to use

Baths, compresses, massage affected area

Circulatory Problems

The most obvious symptom of poor circulation is cold hands and feet, although there may be a general feeling of coldness, which is not necessarily relieved by exercise. Sometimes the lips and extremities actually turn blue. Medical advice should be sought if the poor circulation is associated with atherosclerosis and heart problems.

Essential oils can boost the blood circulation and help to prevent other circulatory problems such as hemorrhoids, cellulite, broken capillaries, and varicose veins.

Once again, diet is important. Foods should be rich in vitamin C, bioflavonoids, and vitamin E. Getting plenty of exercise is also important.

Oils to use

Cypress, neroli, lemon, rose

How to use

Massage, baths

✿ COLDS

Colds tend to attack when you are tired or run down. They are more common in winter because of a lack of fresh foods and a greater consumption of starchy foods. There are many varieties of cold viruses, all of which can easily be caught through coughing, sneezing, and hand contact.

There is no cure for the cold but there are a number of measures you can take to ensure prevention or, once caught, to hasten the cold's departure and relieve your symptoms. Consume as much fruit and vegetables as you can. Make sure you are getting plenty of vitamin C—in supplement form if necessary.

Oils to use

Cinnamon, eucalyptus, niaouli, pine, clove, tea tree, geranium, thyme, cajeput, basil, lavender

How to use

Room spray, baths, chest rubs, inhalation, rub around nose, gargle

✿ COLD SORES

Cold sores are caused by the herpes simplex virus. Once caught, this virus remains in the nervous system and can re-emerge if the immune system is under stress—usually when we are exhausted or if we have been exposed to excess heat or cold. The sores are blister-like in appearance and are first felt—rather than seen—tingling and itching. The blisters are located around the mouth and may last for a week or so. It is difficult to treat the condition.

It is important to build up the immune system through a good diet. Essential oils can help to relieve the symptoms rather than provide a cure.

Oils to use

Eucalyptus, tea tree, chamomile

How to use

Dab on with cotton wool

✺ COLIC

Colic is usually associated with crying babies but it can also occur in adults. In infants it is thought to be caused by air or gas trapped in the immature intestines, which results in pain; the baby may draw his or her legs up when experiencing a spasm. Some authorities believe that allergy to cow's milk is the main reason for the discomfort and it is true that breastfed babies suffer less than bottle-fed babies. In adults, colic is experienced as acute abdominal pains, particularly after eating. Remember do not use any oils on infants without first consulting a professional health care practitioner.

Oils to use

Melissa, chamomile, fennel, caraway

How to use

Baths, massage, rub abdomen with massage oil

✺ COLITIS

This term covers a number of conditions, all of which involve inflammation of the colon—irritable bowel syndrome and ulcerative colitis are the two most common. Colitis can be triggered by stress, anxiety, food intolerance, and bacterial infection. Symptoms include diarrhea, possibly stained with blood, and pain in the lower abdomen.

It is important to seek medical advice. The diet may have to be adjusted by eliminating wheat and dairy products. Food should be cooked well. Drink plenty of fluids.

Oils to use

Chamomile

How to use

Baths, massage

✖ COUGHS

Coughs usually go together with colds, but can also be caused by nervousness, environmental irritants, hay fever, sore throats, asthma, and tonsillitis. The purpose of a cough is to rid the lungs of an irritant—usually excess mucus. Try to keep indoors as much as possible in order to avoid spreading germs through coughing. Stay warm.

Oils to use

Rose, hyssop, eucalyptus, geranium, ginger, lavender, lemon, sandalwood

How to use

Baths, steam inhalation, rub on chest

✖ CRAMPS

A cramp involves a sudden painful contraction of muscle, which mostly occurs in the calves and the feet, most commonly at night. Pregnant women are prone to them during the last three months of pregnancy, as are anemic young women or women who suffer from painful menstruation.

Self-help measures include bending the knee as far as it will go; standing at arm's length from a wall, placing the palms of your hands flat against the wall and leaning into it with feet flat on the floor. If you suffer from stomach cramps, heat is a good remedy. Supplementation with calcium and magnesium can help generally as well as consuming calcium-rich foods, such as green leafy vegetables.

Oils to use

Rosemary, geranium, chamomile, juniper, lavender

How to use

Massage, rub affected area with massage oil, baths, poultices

Cuts

With minor cuts, medical attention usually is not needed. Exceptions are when infection sets in or if the cause was something rusty or dirty, or when the wound is deep and a lot of blood is flowing. In about two hours the clotting factors in the blood will have sealed over the wound.

Essential oils can help to keep the area sterile and to stimulate the production of new skin cells. Most oils also have antibacterial properties. Before you apply any treatment you should wash the wound with clean swabs.

Oils to use

Eucalyptus, lavender, geranium, clary sage, tea tree, chamomile, rose

How to use

On swabs to cleanse, compresses, dab drops on cotton wool and apply

Cystitis

This is usually regarded as a women's complaint although it is possible for men to suffer, too. Women suffer more frequently from cystitis because the female urethra is shorter than the male's and is situated closer to the anus. Cystitis is an infection caused by bacteria entering the bladder through the urethra. Urination is painful and frequent. If not treated in time, the infection can spread right up to the kidneys. If blood appears in the urine, if you are suffering also from a low back pain and have a fever, or if you are pregnant, you should consult a doctor.

Those especially susceptible to cystitis are women on the pill, pregnant women, and newly sexually active women.

Oils to use

Eucalyptus, juniper, lavender, sandalwood, cajeput, pine

How to use

Baths, bidets, massage, hot and cold compresses, rub abdomen with massage oil

✤ DANDRUFF

People with overactive sebaceous glands often suffer from dandruff, which is the excessive shedding of scales of dead skin from the scalp. Sometimes bacteria or fungus are present, too. Poor diet is linked to this disorder, as are emotional and hormonal upsets. Harsh medicated shampoos can sometimes make the condition worse; it is better to use a mild one like a baby shampoo. It is useful to rub the scalp with herbal infusions of burdock, nettles, rosemary, or thyme, especially between shampoos.

Oils to use

Patchouli, cypress, cedarwood, rosemary, mandarin orange

How to use

Scalp massage, hair tonics, rinses

✤ DEPRESSION

Most of us feel depressed at some time or other, perhaps due to a bereavement, loss of a job, the break-up of a relationship, money worries, health problems, or difficult living conditions. In time most of us recuperate and get on with living but if the depression is prolonged, then the possible causes need to be investigated. For example, food intolerance can cause depression, as can vitamin and mineral deficiencies and hormonal imbalances. For some people, depression is seasonal and occurs as winter approaches. Where the problem is not straightforward, it is necessary to consult a professional. Counseling and nutritional therapy can help. Fresh air and exercise can also help to lift the spirits. Many essential oils help to balance, relax, and uplift, especially the citrus oils.

Oils to use

Bergamot, jasmine, lavender, sandalwood, mandarin orange, ylang-ylang, basil, marjoram, thyme

How to use

Baths, inhalation, room fragrances, massage

✤ DERMATITIS (SEE ALSO ECZEMA)

This skin condition is similar to eczema in that its symptoms also include inflammation, swelling, itchy rashes, blisters, and weeping scabs. The skin may become flaky and thick. There are several forms of dermatitis, each with a different cause. Sometimes it may be triggered by dairy products or wheat. Or it may be the skin's response to some sort of chemical such as those found in soap or antiperspirant. Stress or exhaustion can also be responsible for it flaring up.

Oils to use

Chamomile, cypress, fennel, frankincense, geranium, hyssop, juniper, lavender, patchouli, sandalwood

How to use

Baths, compresses, apply diluted oil to the affected area. See chapter 8 on skin care.

✤ DIARRHEA

Diarrhea is the body's way of trying to get rid of an irritant in the bowel. It can be caused by infection, food poisoning, stress, fear, antibiotics, and other drugs. Sometimes it is symptomatic of something more serious, such as Crohn's disease or colitis.

Diarrhea is particularly serious in babies and the elderly and care must be taken to ensure that they do not become dehydrated. They need to be given plenty of fluids. Solid food should be avoided for a couple of days. When the diarrhea has stopped, you can start eating cooked vegetables, soups, and fruit again. White rice is good for helping to stop diarrhea and live yogurt helps to get the friendly bacteria in the intestines back to normal.

Oils to use

Chamomile, eucalyptus, geranium, lavender, lemon, peppermint, rosemary, sandalwood

How to use

Compresses, massage, poultices

Earache

This complaint is common in young children, particularly during or after a cold or flu when there is likely to be catarrhal congestion. This is because the eustachian tube in children's ears is short and easily blocked. The pain is caused by an infection or an inflammation in the middle or outer ear. Other symptoms may include a fever or partial deafness. Sometimes the earache is symptomatic of dental decay or teething or it could mean the start of mumps. Medical advice should be sought if the problem keeps reappearing, if there is bleeding or a discharge, if the eardrum is perforated, or the pain is accompanied by a fever.

Self-help measures include hot salt packs or a covered hot-water bottle held against the ear. Be sure to consult with a professional before treating young children.

Oils to use

Lavender, myrrh, chamomile, clove, geranium

How to use

Cotton ball dabbed with massage oil and placed in ear

❧ ECZEMA (SEE ALSO DERMATITIS)

Like dermatitis the skin becomes inflamed, itchy, red, and swollen. The causes can be external, such as detergents or skin-care products. Or they can be internal, such as occurs in families with a history of allergies, or where the individual is stressed or fatigued. Because it is hard not to scratch the rash, care must be taken to ensure that the area does not become infected. The condition is a complex one and it is best to seek expert advice.

Oils to use

Chamomile, fennel, frankincense, geranium, hyssop, juniper, lavender, sandalwood,

How to use

Baths, apply massage oil to affected areas after patch test

❧ EDEMA (SEE FLUID RETENTION)

❧ EXHAUSTION

If you are suffering from exhaustion, it may be due to a number of factors, such as emotional upheaval, problems in the workplace, or doing too much in too short a space of time. Hormonal changes can also be responsible for feelings of exhaustion, particularly in puberty, pregnancy, and menopause. If you are feeling completely lethargic and it is an ongoing condition, you should consult a doctor to be sure that there is nothing serious underlying it. Essential oils can help you to relax and revitalize.

Oils to use

Clary sage, neroli, lavender, chamomile, basil, orange, bergamot, lemon, thyme, frankincense

How to use

Baths, massage, room fragrance

✂ FEVER

Most of us panic when our children come down with a fever, but in most instances there is no cause for concern. Fever (a body temperature two or more degrees above the norm of 98.6 degrees F) is actually the body's way of helping to destroy invading organisms that are responsible for infections. Thus a fever shouldn't be suppressed unless it becomes dangerously high. The fever may be accompanied by sweating and feeling hot—the body's way of clearing out the toxins and regulating the temperature—or there may be chills and shivering.

A fever lasting more than two days should be brought to medical attention. So should one that cannot be brought under control, or where the patient is a young child.

If the temperature goes up to 40 degrees C (104 degree F) you will need to take action to cool the body down with either a tepid bath or a sponge-bath with tepid water.

Oils to use

Eucalyptus, lavender, lemongrass, rosemary, tea tree, chamomile, clove, coriander, cypress, thyme

How to use

Baths; neck, hand, and foot massage

✂ FLATULENCE

Otherwise known as "gas," flatulence occurs when the stomach and intestines are distended by inhaled air or bacterial activity that produces gas. If we are nervous or anxious we tend to gasp more and thus swallow more air than normal. The other cause of gas is the consumption of foods that contain sugars which then ferment, such as beans, green peppers, and cabbage. Some people have problems digesting their food, which can also cause flatulence.

Use herbs and spices such as mint, fennel seeds, and licorice in cooking to aid digestion. Chewing angelica stems after a meal can help.

Oils to use

Chamomile, fennel, peppermint, basil, rosemary, mandarin orange, cardamom, clove, laurel, lemongrass, marjoram

How to use

Massage abdomen

𝒳 Flu

Flu is the result of a viral infection, which often occurs in epidemics because it is highly contagious. Generally it is not particularly dangerous, except to the elderly or those with heart or lung problems.

The main symptoms are aching muscles and back, fever, headaches, shivering, sweating, coughs, sore throat, catarrh, sneezing, chest pains, and weakness. It is usually over within a week.

Heavy sweating means loss of fluids so it is important to drink plenty of natural liquids. Stay in bed and keep warm. You will do no one at work any favors by showing up sick.

Oils to use

Eucalyptus, fennel, frankincense, ginger, peppermint

How to use

Baths, compresses, massage, inhalation

𝒳 Fluid Retention (Edema)

Where excess fluid is retained in the body, the tissues may swell or puff up, usually around the hands, feet, or eyes. The most common site is the ankles because gravity draws the fluid down. In women, pregnancy, the pill, and premenstrual hormones are the usual causes of fluid retention. Allergic reactions, standing or sitting for prolonged periods, and injury can also cause edema.

Oils to use

Eucalyptus, chamomile, lavender, rosemary, cypress, lemon, wintergreen

How to use

Baths; massage legs, hands, soles of the feet, abdomen, and solar plexus; compresses

FRIGIDITY

Most sexual problems are not long-term ones and can be helped effectively by aromatherapy—especially those that are related to depression, stress, and anxiety, all of which hinder the sexual response. Massage with essential oils can be a particularly good way of helping partners to relax and to build up their relationship. Some people swear by the aphrodisiac properties of certain oils. If the problem is not short term, however, counseling may be needed.

Oils to use

Clary sage, neroli, patchouli, rose, sandalwood, ylang-ylang

How to use

Baths, massage, room fragrance

GINGIVITIS (SEE GUM DISEASE)

GOUT

Uric acid builds up in the joints when the kidneys are unable to excrete it properly. The acid is deposited in the form of crystals, which then restrict the movement of the joints, causing inflammation. Gout is normally manifested in the big toe, although other joints can be affected. It can be extremely painful. It is usually brought on by alcohol, drugs, an overindulgent diet, and even surgery. It tends to afflict men more than women

Obesity and a diet overly high in protein increases your chances of getting gout. Your diet may need to be adjusted to include foods that help the kidneys to excrete the uric acid. These include carrots, celery, tomatoes, leeks, and onions. Fats and red meat should be avoided.

Oils to use

Pine, rosemary, juniper, tea tree, cajeput, frankincense

How to use

Foot baths, massage, compresses

✻ GRIEF

Profound emotional pain can strike with devastating consequences and can last months or even years. Grief can weaken the immune system, opening the door for a variety of ailments. Essential oils lift the spirits and strengthen the immune system.

Oils to use

Cypress, frankincense, marjoram, rose, mandarin orange

How to use

Baths, massage, room fragrance

✻ GUM DISEASE

You can avoid gum infections by regular brushing and flossing, avoiding sugar, and eating a good diet with plenty of fresh fruit and vegetables rich in vitamin C.

Gum disease is also known as gingivitis and its symptoms are swollen, bleeding, and infected gums. If it is left untreated, the individual can develop more serious disorders that undermine the immune system. Loss of teeth is one of the major consequences.

Pregnancy can trigger gingivitis, as can other hormonal changes such as puberty, menopause, or taking an oral contraceptive pill.

Oils to use

Cypress, lemon, tea tree, thyme, clove, clary sage

How to use

Mouthwash, rub onto gums

✻ HAIR LOSS (ALOPECIA)

Baldness, especially in men, is usually attributed to genetic factors that come into play depending on age and hormonal changes. However, it can be exacerbated by other conditions such as stress, shock, scalp conditions (dandruff, eczema, etc.), and poor diet. In women, it may be caused by overuse of hair products and treatments, or by pregnancy. Some drug therapies can cause baldness. The loss of hair can be total, partial, or patchy.

Massage with essential oils can be beneficial because it helps to stimulate the skin and the hair follicles.

Oils to use

Lavender, rosemary, ylang-ylang

How to use

Massage scalp

Hangover

A long, hot bath with essential oil of juniper or pepper can be especially soothing.

Oils to use

Juniper, pepper, rose, rosemary

How to use

Baths, inhalation, massage

Hay Fever

When summer arrives many people respond by sneezing. That, together with a runny nose and red eyes, is one of the major symptoms of hay fever. Essentially, it is a chronic allergic reaction, mainly to pollen but also to dust, chemicals, and smoke. The predisposition toward hay fever is usually inherited. Other members of the family may suffer from eczema or asthma. Sometimes hay fever can be triggered by a food intolerance—such as to dairy products or wheat. Herbal teas such as fenugreek and vitamin C supplements can be beneficial.

Oils to use

Eucalyptus, cajeput, tea tree, juniper

How to use

Gargles, inhalations, chest rubs, a few drops on a handkerchief, room fragrance

❧ HEADACHES (SEE ALSO COLDS, FLU, HANGOVER)

There are many causes of headaches—among them, stress, allergies, high blood pressure, muscle tension, and infections such as colds and flu. Some women suffer from headaches when they are premenstrual. Cold wind or a hot, stuffy environment can also bring one on.

Headaches caused by stress or muscle tension are particularly well-suited to massage with essential oils. Compresses over the eyes are soothing. If the headache is due to congestion, then inhalations are best.

Oils to use

Clary sage, chamomile, lavender, marjoram, rose, peppermint, rosemary, basil, melissa, cajeput, tea tree, juniper, pepper

How to use

Compresses; massage with oil the head, neck, and shoulders; baths; room fragrance

❧ HEMORRHOIDS

Hemorrhoids are caused by distended veins in either the anal canal or around the rectum. They can be caused by excessive straining to pass stools, especially when constipated. Incorrect lifting of heavy weights can also put pressure on the abdominal muscles.

The condition is more often found in overweight or sedentary individuals or in pregnant women. Hemorrhoids can be itchy and bleed. Inflammation and soreness may also be experienced. Severe cases may require surgery, but mostly hemorrhoids can be cured with self-treatment.

Oils to use

Myrtle, cypress, frankincense

How to use

Massage, external application of massage oil, sitz baths, baths

✄ HOARSENESS AND LOSS OF VOICE

These conditions can be caused by a variety of factors, such as colds, flu, laryngitis, and tonsillitis. Laryngitis is caused by an inflammation of the larynx, due to a bacterial or viral infection. If it is acute, there can be pain and mucus, although the sufferer will feel as if his or her throat is extremely dry. People who breath through their mouths or who work in a dusty environment may suffer from chronic laryngitis. With tonsillitis, also caused by viruses or bacteria, the tonsils at the back of the throat become inflamed and enlarged and there is difficulty swallowing. Tonsillitis occurs more frequently in children.

Oils to use

Cypress, lavender, sandalwood, tea tree, rose, pepper, myrrh, clary sage

How to use

Baths, inhalation, rub on chest and throat, gargles

✄ HYSTERIA

Caused by tension or excitement, hysteria is characterized by a temporary loss of control over the emotions. Essential oils are helpful in regaining calm and control.

Oils to use

Chamomile, clary sage, lavendar, spikenard

How to use

Baths, room fragrance, massage

❧ IMPETIGO

A disorder that mainly afflicts children, impetigo is caused by *streptococcus* or *staphylococcus* bacteria. The symptoms include inflamed, puffy patches or spots that blister and crust over. These appear mostly on the face, scalp, and neck, and sometimes on the hands and knees. Impetigo is contagious. Antibiotics are the usual form of treatment.

Conditions must be kept hygienic in order to prevent the spread of impetigo. If it is neglected, the results can be serious, especially in adults. If it is on the scalp, hair loss can result.

Essential oils can help by keeping the skin sterilized and relieving any itching.

Oils to use

Benzoin, calendula, chamomile, tea tree

How to use

Apply massage oil to infected areas once a day

❧ IMPOTENCE (SEE FRIGIDITY)

❧ INDIGESTION

Eating too fast is the most common cause of this complaint. We should all take time to eat and digest food without being in a hurry. Digestion is also impaired if we are feeling anxious or angry. Tension impairs the flow of blood to the digestive organs.

It is tempting to rely on antacids to treat the problem, but prolonged use of them can be counterproductive because they cause the body to overcompensate in its manufacturing of stomach acid thereby compounding the problem. Severe pain radiating to your back may indicate that you have a peptic ulcer which needs attention. Foods that can cause indigestion include fried foods, cheese, and onions. Herbal teas such as chamomile or peppermint can help.

Oils to use

Bergamot, chamomile, fennel, juniper, lavender, lemon, peppermint, rosemary, mandarin orange

How to use

Baths, massage, rub abdomen with massage oil

❧ INSOMNIA

Insomnia can either mean finding it difficult to go to sleep or, having fallen asleep, waking early and finding it difficult to go back to sleep. We often suffer from this complaint during times of great stress, change, or hormonal imbalances (for example, during menstruation or menopause). Insomnia is a phenomenon often experienced by the elderly.

One easily spotted cause is excessive intake of stimulants such as coffee, alcohol, or cigarettes. Or it may be that we get too little exercise. It is best to avoid sleeping pills and tranquilizers because an addiction can develop.

To counter insomnia, avoid any stimulants after 4:00 P.M. Melatonin supplements can help or try herbal teas such as chamomile.

Oils to use

Lavender, chamomile, marjoram, orange, rose, sandalwood, ylang-ylang

How to use

Baths, massage, room fragrance, a few drops on a tissue near the pillow

❧ IRRITABILITY

Short-term emotional problems, anxiety over a specific event, or high stress levels can lead to the condition of irritability. Suddenly, even minor things get inflated into major incidents. At these times, nothing is more soothing than a bath or massage using your favorite essential oil. Soon the restorative capacity of the oils will help you put things in perspective.

Oils to use

Chamomile, cypress, lemon, ylang-ylang

How to use

Baths, massage, inhalation, room fragrance

❧ LARYNGITIS (SEE HOARSENESS AND LOSS OF VOICE)

❧ LUMBAGO

More commonly known as backache, the symptoms are severe pain in the lower back. Lumbago is mostly caused by incorrect lifting of heavy objects or by having twisted the spine in an awkward position. Some women experience it in pregnancy. Often, the sufferer cannot stand straight again for a few moments after stooping. Good ways to relieve the symptoms are to have adequate bed rest, heat, and massage. Hot baths can help.

Oils to use

Rosemary thyme, juniper, pine

How to use

Baths, poultices, massage

❧ LOSS OF APPETITE (SEE ALSO ANOREXIA)

Oils to use

Bergamot, chamomile, fennel, peppermint

How to use

Baths, compresses, massage, room fragrance

❧ MEMORY (POOR)

As we become older, most of us feel a diminished ability to retain and recall information, ideas, and impressions. Many factors contribute to this condition, not just aging. Essential oils can help by soothing and calming the nerves.

Oils to use

Basil, juniper, rosemary

How to use

Baths, inhalation, massage

Menopause

Although all women go through menopause, it is often approached with fear. However, menopause is just another phase in a woman's life, and for many women it is a time of liberation and fulfillment. It usually occurs between the ages of forty-five and fifty and involves the cessation of menstruation—sometimes suddenly, usually gradually—and a reduction in production of certain hormones, primarily estrogen.

Some women suffer to a greater or lesser extent from a variety of symptoms, which include hot flashes, night sweating, mental depression, anxiety, vaginal discomfort, itchy skin, irritability, and lack of sexual desire (although the opposite has been reported!). Fear can actually exacerbate the symptoms.

Herbal teas such as chamomile are beneficial because they can help to tone the relevant areas of the body; some of them have properties that act in similar ways to the female hormones.

Exercise can play a part in relaxation. Have a regular massage. Avoid stimulants.

Oils to use

Chamomile, rosemary, thyme, lavender, sandalwood, melissa, cypress, cardamom

How to use

Baths, massage, inhalation

Menstruation

Most women, at some time in their lives, will experience an upset in their menstrual cycle. Perhaps their period is unusually heavy, or it has been delayed for a few days, or has become irregular. Many women suffer severe pain just before their period, with some having to take to their beds with a hot-water bottle. These upsets are often caused by hormonal imbalances. Sometimes emotional crises will affect the pattern.

Conventional treatment has been to offer diuretics, tranquilizers, or the oral contraceptive pill. What these do not do, however, is to rebalance the hypothalamus and the pituitary gland, which are the two parts of the body that regulate the menstrual cycle through the release of hormones. Essential oils are very beneficial for treating menstrual problems, perhaps because some plant essences help normalize hormone secretions by stimulating the endocrine glands.

Oils to use

Heavy periods—Cypress
Irregular periods—Chamomile, geranium
Painful menstruation—Clary sage, juniper, rosemary

How to use

Baths, compresses, rub abdomen with massage oil

✻ Mental Fatigue

A little stress is good for you, but being under constant stress leads to a state of mental fatigue, where you are drained not physically, but emotionally. Meditation and other forms of relaxation can help. Essential oils can complement that process.

Oils to use

Basil, rosemary

How to use

Baths, massage, room fragrance

✻ Mood Swings

We all go through cycles. At times we are happy and at other times we can hardly drag through the day. Diet, work patterns, and high stress levels all contribute to the ups and downs. The pharmaceutical industry offers a multitude of drugs to deal with mood swings. Unfortunately, most of these drugs are dangerous and many have undesirable side effects. Essential oils can offer a much more pleasant and rational alternative to prescription drugs.

Oils to use

Eucalyptus, chamomile, geranium, lavender

How to use

Baths, massage, room fragrance

Motion Sickness (See Nausea)

Nausea

Nausea can be caused by strong emotions—nervousness, fear, revulsion—or something physical, such as pregnancy or an infection. Food allergies can bring on nausea as can traveling. If you feel sick, it is better not to eat, although some people find toast and plain white rice helpful. Fresh air can be of benefit if the sickness is caused by motion. Herbal teas, especially mint, may alleviate the symptoms.

Oils to use

Fennel, lavender, peppermint

How to use

Baths, inhalation

Nervous Tension (See Also Anxiety, Stress)

Oils to use

Cypress, marjoram, rose, sandalwood, mandarin orange, ylang-ylang

How to use

Baths, massage, room fragrance

❧ NEURALGIA

Neuralgia is pain caused by an inflamed or compressed nerve sheath. The stabbing or burning pain usually is felt in the face. Neuralgia is not a disease in its own right but is rather a symptom of another disorder such as toothache, sinusitis, shingles, migraine, or a slipped disc, making it necessary to treat the underlying cause. This may necessitate a visit to a chiropractor or osteopath if there is any misalignment of the neck and back. Herbal teas can be used to help the sufferer relax, or try soothing yourself by using the oils listed below.

Oils to use

Pepper, chamomile, eucalyptus, geranium, lemon, tea tree, peppermint

How to use

Baths, compresses, rub affected area with massage oil

❧ OBSESSIONS

It is best to seek counseling if you are suffering from an obsession so that you can identify the reasons giving rise to that behavior. In conjunction with expert help, essential oils can help you to relax and to lay those obsessions aside for a while. Massage will, through the medium of touch, help to make you feel cared for and connected with another human being.

Oils to use

Clary sage, frankincense

How to use

Baths, inhalation, massage

❧ PREMENSTRUAL TENSION

Just before menstruation, many women suffer from a range of physical and emotional symptoms. They may gain weight, feel bloated, suffer stomach cramps and sore breasts, be unable to sleep, and break out in acne. Often they will feel lethargic or irritable and tearful. The cause of all these ailments appears to be an imbalance in the levels of the hormones estrogen and progesterone, which are controlled by the hypothalamus and the pituitary gland. Relaxing with essential oils will help to bring these hormones back into balance. Evening primrose oil is renowned for easing the symptoms of premenstrual tension.

Oils to use

Chamomile, cypress, geranium, lavender, rose, pine, neroli

How to use

Baths, compresses, massage

Psoriasis

The symptoms of this skin condition include circular patches of reddened or pink skin, which may be covered with dry, silvery-white, flaky skin. These patches are found mainly on the forehead, knees, and elbows. It is possible for the lesions to become pustular. The nails and the inside of the ear can also become affected. Psoriasis is extremely itchy. Often it disappears, only to reappear at a later time.

Psoriasis is caused by a faulty immune system, which overproduces skin cells; anxiety and stress can trigger its appearance. It has been linked to rheumatoid arthritis. Treatment is usually long term because the disease is complex. Diet may need adjusting to exclude foods that contain caffeine.

Oils to use

Bergamot, benzoin, geranium, cajeput, lavender, juniper, tea tree

How to use

Baths, compresses, massage oil applied to affected areas

❧ RHEUMATISM

This condition involves inflammation of the joints and muscles. There may be stiffness, too. Rheumatism is really a catch-all term to describe a number of ailments, including arthritis and fibrositis, with a variety of possible causes.

The underlying factors should be addressed and it is best to see a practitioner for this. Modification of diet may help. Reduce consumption of dairy products and wheat and avoid coffee, tea, red meat, sugar, and refined and processed foods. Also try to avoid foods that contain oxalic acid such as alfalfa and rhubarb. Fish oils are beneficial. Essential oils can help by enhancing the immune system and reducing inflammation.

Oils to use

Chamomile, eucalyptus, lavender, lemon, marjoram, rosemary, wintergreen

How to use

Baths, compresses, massage affected area with massage oil

❧ SHOCK

Be it a reaction to bad news or an accident, the body reacts by going into a state of shock. Both physical and emotional shock symptoms can be mitigated by the use of essential oils.

Oils to use

Neroli, melissa, peppermint, rose, ylang-ylang

How to use

Baths, massage, room fragrance

❧ SHINGLES

Shingles are caused by the same virus that is responsible for chicken pox. It lies dormant in the body and then reappears when you are run down. Only those people who have had chicken pox can get shingles. Part of a nerve becomes infected with the virus, which then reappears during times of stress. There may be a fever and a rash of small blisters develops, running along a set of nerves. There is also sometimes severe, stabbing pain, which can continue long after the rash has disappeared. Shingles can appear on the face and the blisters can damage the sight if located near the eyes. Consult a doctor if this is the case. Essential oils can help treat shingles by enhancing immune function and improving blood circulation under the skin.

Oils to use

Geranium, lavender, myrtle, rosemary (in combination or singly)

How to use

Massage affected area

Sinusitis

With sinusitis, the sinuses are congested with mucus and the tissues of the sinus passages have become infected and inflamed. The symptoms include fatigue, nose bleeds, nasal congestion, headaches, ear pain, and pain around the eyes. There may also be a mild fever accompanied by a cough. Apart from its association with complications of a cold, sinusitis may also be due to insufficient vitamin A. Cold and damp may be exacerbating factors.

Oils to use

Benzoin, cajeput, tea tree, lavender, eucalyptus, basil

How to use

Baths, inhalation, compresses

Skin Problems (See Acne, Chilblains, Eczema, Psoriasis, Sunburn, and Chapter 8)

❧ STIFFNESS (SEE ALSO RHEUMATISM, STRESS)

Much of the stiffness in our joints can be attributed to lack of exercise. However, other factors may cause or contribute to the problem, including old age, rheumatic disorders, emotional problems, stress, and damp and cold weather. Exercise is an obvious way of countering the condition. Hot baths with essential oils are particularly helpful.

Oils to use

Eucalyptus, lavender, rosemary, pine, marjoram, cajeput

How to use

Baths, massage, compresses

❧ STOMACHACHE (SEE ALSO INDIGESTION)

Stomachaches can be the result of a number of unpleasant digestive ailments and are often accompanied by bloating, diarrhea, heartburn, and gas. Licorice and anise seeds have long been recognized as effective treatments.

Oils to use

Fennel, lavender, marjoram, peppermint, rosemary

How to use

Baths, massage abdomen

❧ STRESS

Stress is a natural part of life. It is overwhelming, excessive stress that is damaging. When adrenaline is being constantly produced, it can interfere with the way our bodies function—even causing serious health problems such as high blood pressure. It is generally considered that modern times are stressful times, although others have argued that the famines, floods, and disease experienced by our ancestors cannot have been anything other than stressful.

Symptoms of stress include impaired digestion, insomnia, irritability, fatigue, depression, and lack of resistance to viral and bacterial infections.

Self-help measures include counseling, yoga, exercise, and giving yourself some positive strokes. Essential oils can help to relax you and make you feel pampered.

Oils to use

Basil, lavender, marjoram, melissa, orange, clary sage, ylang-ylang

How to use

Baths, massage, room fragrance

✂ SUNBURN

Fair-skinned people are especially prone to sunburn because they have little melanin in their skin, which causes pigmentation and protects skin from ultraviolet rays. If the sunburn is minor, there is usually some reddening of the skin and some discomfort, which may be followed by a tan. If the sunburn is more serious, then the skin and tissues swell considerably and the pain is intense. The skin can blister and peel.

Skin cancer, caused by sunbathing, is on the increase. The sun can also make the skin tough and wrinkled. Try to avoid sunbathing for prolonged periods, use a sunscreen, and if you do become sunburned, wait for the skin to cool down before applying any lotions.

Oils to use

Lavender

How to use

Baths, cold compresses; add 2 drops to a cup of natural yogurt and apply

✂ TONSILLITIS (SEE HOARSENESS AND LOSS OF VOICE)

✀ Toothaches

In an adult, tooth pain is usually associated with an infection or dental decay. The oils below can be soothing and help fight an infection.

Oils to use

Chamomile, clove, peppermint

How to use

Mouthwash, compresses

✀ Urinary Infections (See Cystitis)

✀ Varicose Veins (See Also Chapter 7)

Whether we develop varicose veins depends to some extent on heredity. In women they often occur during pregnancy, usually in the legs because of the effects of gravity. Blood collects in the veins, which then swell up and twist. The legs often ache and the veins may itch. People who stand a lot have a tendency to develop this condition, particularly if they are also overweight or constipated.

Try to avoid standing for long periods and try to lie down with your feet raised above the level of your heart. Don't sit cross-legged. Get plenty of exercise. Ice packs can help. Essential oils can help by improving circulation; they also have anti-inflammatory and anti-coagulating properties.

Oils to use

Cypress, lavender, lemon

How to use

Baths, compresses, massage

✤ WARTS (VERRUCAE)

Warts are caused by a virus, which produces the unsightly skin growths. They are contagious and usually manifest themselves when we are run down. It may be necessary to check for underlying causes. A mixture of raw garlic and onion applied to the wart overnight is supposed to help remove warts. Lemon and tea tree essential oils will enhance the immune system and thus help it to fight off the virus.

Oils to use

Lemon, tea tree

How to use

Dab wart with oil

✤ WOUNDS AND SORES (SEE ALSO CUTS)

With minor cuts, the damaged blood vessels slowly contract, stopping the flow of blood. Then a clot forms to plug the wound. As the skin around the cut regenerates, the scab gets smaller and smaller until the wound disappears. Essential oils can speed up the process of healing and help to minimize scarring.

Oils to use

Lavender, patchouli

How to use

Baths, compresses

Useful Contacts

To obtain a reference for a qualified aromatherapist, or to learn more about aromatherapy resources in your area, contact the following:

American Alliance of Aromatherapy
P.O. Box 750428
Petaluma, CA 94975

Canadian Federation of Aromatherapists
868 Markham Road
Suite 109
Scarborough, ON
Canada M1H 2Y2
416-439-1951

International Federation of Aromatherapists
2–4 Chiswick High Road
London W4 England
0181-742-2605

National Assocation for Holistic Aromatherapy
P.O. Box 17622
Boulder, CO 80308-7622
800-566-6735

Glossary

Absolute   Extract from plant material, usually flowers, that is obtained by using solvents such as benzene or hexane.

Analgesic   A painkiller; some essential oils contain analgesic properties.

Antispasmodic   Capable of preventing and relieving spasms, convulsions, nervous disorders.

Carminitive   Expels gas to relieve flatulence or colic.

Colic   Severe spasmodic pain in the stomach, occurring in waves of increased intensity.

Concrete   Product extracted by use of volatile solvents and containing chemical residues from the solvents. Used mainly by the perfume industry.

Cold-press   Method of extracting carrier oils without the use of heat or solvents to ensure high retention of nutrients.

Compress   Wet or dry cloth or gauze pad applied to a part of the body to relieve pain, reduce a fever, drain a wound.

Contusion   An injury where the skin is not broken, such as a bruise.

Decoction   An extract of water-soluble substances from a medicinal plant obtained through boiling.

Depurative   Purifies the blood and other bodily fluids.

Diaphoretic   Promotes perspiration.

Diuretic   A substance that increases the flow of urine.

Emmenagogic   A substance that promotes menstrual discharge.

Essence   A natural aromatic substance secreted by a plant.

Essential oil   A product resulting from the steam distillation of aromatic plants; an essential oil is distilled essence.

Galactagogic   A substance that promotes the flow of breastmilk.

Hemostatic   An agent that slows down or stops bleeding

Hypothalamus   Neural control center at the base of the brain, concerned with hunger, thirst, and other autonomic functions.

Infusion   An extract obtained by soaking plant material in water.

Neat   Pure essential oil undiluted by any carrier oil.

Neuralgic   Counteracts severe spasmodic pain along the course of a nerve.

Note   A measure of the volatility (rate of evaporation) of an essential oil. Top notes are the most volatile and base notes the least.

Pessary   A device placed in the vagina to treat vaginal disorders such as thrush.

Phenol   One of a class of weakly acidic compounds that exert beneficial effects on the liver, skin, and mucous membranes.

Pheromone   A chemical substance secreted by some animals that affects the behavior or physiology of other animals of the same species.

Poultice   Method of applying herbs to the body by adding hot water to a cloth bag filled with plant substances.

Stomachic   A stimulant or tonic for the stomach; digestive aid.

Sudorific   Promotes or causes perspiration.

Tincture   Concentrated extract of either fresh or dried plant substances in a mixture of water and alcohol.

Tisane   A liquid preparation (for drinking) using plant substances.

Vulnerary   Useful in healing wounds.

Selected Bibliography

Auckett, A. 1982. *Baby Massage.* Wellingborough, England: Thorsons.

Buchbauer, G., L. Jirovetz, W. Jager, C. Plank, and H. Dietrich. 1993. Fragrance compounds and essential oils with sedative effects upon inhalation. *Journal of Pharmological Science*, June, v. 82, no. 6: 660–664.

Buning, F., and P. Hambly. 1993. *Herbalism.* London: Headway, Hodder & Stoughton.

Burns, E., and C. Blamey. 1994. Complementary medicine: Using aromatherapy in childbirth. *Nursing Times*, March 2–8, 1994, v. 90, no. 9: 54–60.

Chidell, L. 1992. *Aromatherapy*, 4th ed. London: Headway, Hodder & Stoughton.

Dale, A., and S. Cornwell. 1994. The role of lavender oil in relieving perineal discomfort following childbirth: A blind randomized clinical trial. *Journal of Advanced Nursing*, January, v. 19, no. 1: 89–96.

Dodd, G. H., and M. Skinner. 1992. From moods to molecules: The pyschopharmacology of perfumery and aromatherapy. In *Fragrance: The Psychology and Biology of Perfume*, S. Van Toller and G. H. Dodd, eds. London: Elsevier Science.

Eriksen, M. 1994. Aromatherapy for childbearing. *Mothering*, no. 4 (summer): 74–78.

Fahy, T. A., P. Desilva, P. Silverstone, et al. 1989. The effects of loss of taste and smell in a case of anorexia nervosa and bulimia nervosa. *British Journal of Psychiatry* 155: 860–861.

James, R. 1990. Aromatherapy: The link between good "scents" and good health. *Bestways Magazine*, v. 18, no. 2: 54–55.

Jellinek, J. S. 1991. Odours and perfumes as a system of signs. In *Perfumes: Art, Science, Technology, Applied Science*. London: Elsevier Science.

Kafan, G. 1992. Case studies. *International Journal of Aromatherapy* 4, no. 1 (spring): 33–34.

King, J. R. 1988. Anxiety reduction using fragrances. In *Perfumery: The Psychology and Biology of Fragrance*, S. Van Toller and G. H. Dodd, eds. London: Chapman and Hall.

Lorig, T. S. 1992. Cognitive and non-cognitive effects of odour exposure. In *Fragrance: The Pyschology and Biology of Perfume*, S. Van Toller and G. H. Dodd, eds. London: Elsevier Science.

Mailhebiau, P. 1995. *Portrait in Oils*. Saffron Waldon, England: C W. Daniel.

Mailhebiau, P. (ed.). 1995. Les Cahiers de l'Aromatherapie/Aromatherapy Records, no. 1, Sept. 1995.

Merz. 1989. Scientific Documentation on Balneotherapie, Research and Development Consumer Product Division, Frankfurt.

Paleologos, M. 1990. The power of perfume (psychological effects of fragrances). *Women's Wear Daily*, June 8, 1990, v. 159, no. 112: F78.

Price, S. 1987. *Practical Aromatherapy*, 2nd ed. Wellingborough, England: Thorsons.

Ryan, K. 1988. *Probing Scent Psychology*. New York: Fairchild Publications.

Ryman, D. 1991. *Aromatherapy*. London: Piatkus Books.

Shapiro, D. 1990. *The Bodymind Workbook*. Dorset, England: Element Books.

Stanway, A., ed. 1987. *The Natural Family Doctor*. London: Gaia Books.

Walji, H. 1992. *The Vitamin Guide: Essential Nutrients for Healthy Living*. Dorset, England: Element Books.

———. 1993. *Asthma and Hayfever: Combining Orthodox and Complementary Approaches*. London: Hodder Headline.

———. 1993. *Headaches and Migraines*. London: Hodder Headline.

———. 1993. *Skin Conditions: Orthodox and Complementary Approaches*. London: Hodder Headline.

———. 1994. *Alcohol, Smoking, and Tranquilisers: Orthodox and Complementary Approaches*. London: Hodder Headline.

———. 1994. *Arthritis and Rheumatism: Orthodox and Complementary Approaches*. London: Hodder Headline.

———. 1994. *Heart Health: A Self-Help Guide to Combining Orthodox and Complementary Approaches*. London: Hodder Headline.

———. 1994. *Using Aromatherapy at Home*. Cleaveland, England: CPR Publishing/Holland & Barrett.

———. 1994. *Vitamins, Minerals, and Dietary Supplements: A Definitive Guide to Healthy Eating*. London: Hodder Headline.

Weiss, R. F. 1988. *Herbal Medicine*, 6th ed. Gothenburg, Sweden: AB Arcanum; Beaconsfield, England: Beaconsfield Publishers.

Wildwood, C. 1991. *Aromatherapy: Massage with Essential Oils*. Dorset, England: Element Books.

Index

Page numbers in bold indicate the primary reference.

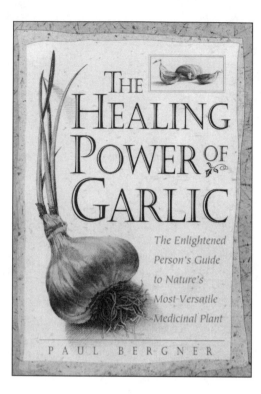

The Healing Power of Garlic

by Paul Bergner

The Healing Power of Garlic explains garlic's historical and contemporary uses and modern science's understanding of how garlic works as a medicine. Paul Bergner, a well-known writer, is editor and publisher of *Medical Herbalism.* He is clinic director at Rocky Mountain Center for Botancial Studies in Boulder, Colorado.
A Selection of the Rodale Book Club

The Healing Power of Ginseng & the Tonic Herbs

by Paul Bergner

Best known of the herbs in the tonic family, ginseng can slowly build up an exhausted and over-stressed system and improve overall energy, strength, and vitality. *The Healing Power of Ginseng and the Tonic Herbs* explores the practical healing uses of ginseng and other powerful tonic herbs.

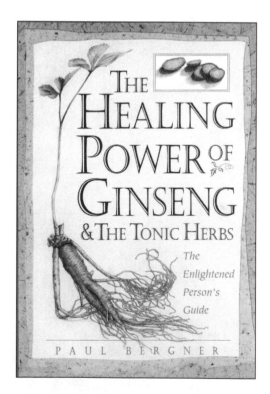

The Healing Power of Herbs

by Michael T. Murray

In this up-to-date and carefully researched book on botancial medicine, Dr. Murray brings you the latest scientific findings about the power and efficacy of medicinal herbs. Michael T. Murray, N.D., is a leading researcher and lecturer in the field of natural medicine. He is author of the bestselling book *The Encyclopedia of Natural Medicine* (Prima).

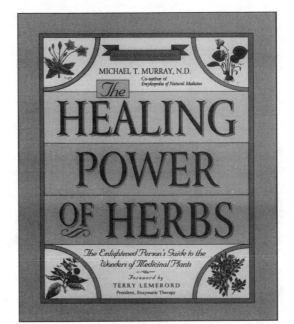

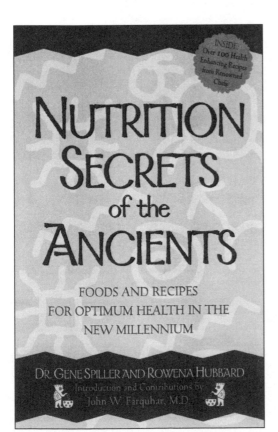

Nutrition Secrets of the Ancients

by Dr. Gene Spiller and Rowena Hubbard

Ancient, natural foods (such as olives, corn, cocoa, yams, and grapes) promote health, weight maintenance, and longevity. This book combines history, science, legends, and more than 100 delicious recipes from world-renowned chefs using these life-enhancing foods. Dr. Gene Spiller wrote *The Superpyramid Eating Program.* He lives in Los Altos, California. Rowena Hubbard is president of Food Resources in Sacramento, California, where she operates a test kitchen.

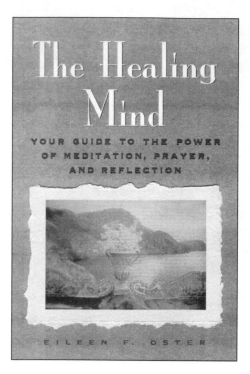

The Healing Mind
by Eileen F. Oster

The strong connection between spiritual, physical, and mental health is widely acknowledged, but few books offer the kind of practical, reader-focused approach provided by Eileen Oster. Her book is designed to help people suffering from long-term illnesses or facing life-threatening diseases. With guided meditations, suggested prayer formats, and visualizations, *The Healing Mind* evolves into the perfect tool for readers hoping to explore the spirit–mind–body connection for overall health and well-being.

Herbal Prescriptions for Better Health
by Donald J. Brown

Herbs such as aloe vera, cayenne, *dong quai,* feverfew, garlic, ginseng, goldenseal, hawthorn, and senna have been used for centuries to cure or control a wide range of medical conditions, but few people know exactly how to administer them. Comprehensive, easy to follow, and organized according to the medical diagnosis, this book will help. Donald J. Brown, N.D., is founder and director of the Natural Products Research Consultants and edits the *Quarterly Review of Natural Medicine.*

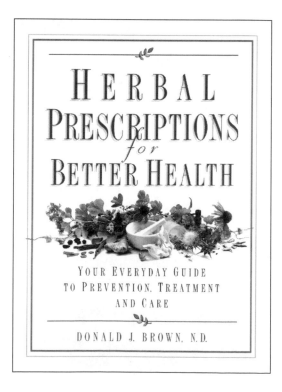

PRIMA PUBLISHING
P.O. Box 1260BK   Rocklin, CA 95677

USE YOUR VISA/MC AND ORDER BY PHONE
(916) 632-4400
Monday–Friday 9 A.M.–4 P.M. PST

I'd like to order copies of the following titles:

Quantity	Title	Amount
_____	_____	_____
_____	_____	_____
_____	_____	_____

Subtotal _____

Postage & Handling* _____

Sales Tax: 7.25% (CA); 5% (IN and MD); 8.25% (TN) _____

TOTAL (U.S. funds only) _____

Check enclosed for $_____(payable to Prima Publishing)

HAWAII, ALASKA, CANADA, FOREIGN, AND PRIORITY REQUEST ORDERS,
PLEASE CALL ORDER ENTRY FOR PRICE QUOTE (916) 632-4400

Charge my   ❑ MasterCard   ❑ Visa

Account No. _____ Exp. Date_____

Print Your Name _____

Your Signature _____

Address _____

City/State/Zip _____

Daytime Telephone (___)_____

*Postage & Handling	
Purchase Amount:	Add:
$14.99 or less..........$3.00	
$15–$29.99 ....$4.00	
$30–$49.99 ....$6.00	
$50–$99.99 ....$10.00	
$100 –$199.99 ......$13.50	

Prices are subject to change.

Please allow three to four weeks for delivery.